THE SENSES

THE SENSES

by Wolfgang von Buddenbrock

ANN ARBOR

THE UNIVERSITY OF MICHIGAN PRESS

Third printing 1962

Published in the United States of America by
The University of Michigan Press and simultaneously
in Toronto, Canada, by Ambassador Books Limited

Library of Congress Catalog Card No. 58-5907

First published as Die Welt der Sinne
Second revised edition 1953 by Springer-Verlag
Berlin–Göttingen–Heidelberg

Translated by Frank Gaynor
Designed by George Lenox

Manufactured in the United States of America

Contents

1657392

THE SENSES

PART ONE

The Senses—Stimulus and Response

1. The Animal and the Outside World

The world we live in is the playground of an infinite number of forces. As you sit by your radio on a quiet evening, listening to music brought to you from far away, you realize that you live in the midst of a vast and intricate network of electromagnetic waves that radiate about you and even right through you. They are everywhere, but without your radio you would never become aware of a certain range of them. Of course radio waves are not natural phenomena, but the radio will also reveal to you the presence of some natural forces. Whenever it crackles, gurgles, and rattles you know that some electric discharge in the air is interfering with the music. Such discharges must have been taking place ever since the day of creation, but a human being who relied solely on his own natural senses would never be aware of their existence.

Our eyes give further testimony of the limitations of the human senses. Electromagnetic waves come in a wide variety of sizes, ranging in a continuous series from the mile-long radio waves to the unbelievably tiny wave lengths of ultraviolet radiation. Our eyes, however, register only a very narrow range—roughly waves of between 800 and 390 millimicrons in length. (One millimicron is 1/1,000,000 millimeter, or 1/25,000,000 inch.) All other radiation is invisible to us.

Our sense of hearing, too, is hemmed in by insurmountable barriers. We can hear no sound, strong as it may be, that vibrates fewer than fifteen or more than 20,000 times a second. These examples—and a great many more could easily be found—illustrate the limitations of our senses. We see that there are two different worlds: the big, objective physical world which the physicists measure and weigh with their instruments, and the subjective world defined by the range of the senses; this latter is what we call the "outside world."

To study the relationship between the physical world and any given form of life, we need only look at a small part of the world surrounding the organism. This part of the physical world is the environment of the particular form of life. Since the environment contains every existing force, the environment of all creatures living at the same place is the same. Furthermore, since a creature's outside world is only a small part of its environment, it follows that the outside world changes with the environment. When a migratory bird flies from a northern to a southern climate, its environment—and along with it everything that the bird perceives—changes considerably. Even more important is the fact that within the same environment different creatures have different outside worlds, depending on the evolutionary level of the creature. Each form of life has its unique outside world.

A simple example will make this clear. Two completely different creatures, a bird and a caterpillar, are perched on a branch of a tree. Both have the same environment, but each lives in its private outside world. The bird keeps glancing about with its keen little eyes. Nothing that takes place on the highway or in the nearby field escapes its watchful attention. It sees the bird of prey that circles high in the sky, and the tiny field mouse that rustles in the foliage below. The caterpillar, however, is unaware of all this activity. Nature has given the caterpillar a few small, quite rudimentary eyes, which can do little more than determine the direction from which the rays of the sun are coming, and whether the day is bright or cloudy. Moreover, the caterpillar is totally deaf, whereas for the bird the air is filled with voices, among them the call of his own kind. The bird, on the other hand, is oblivious of certain distinctions that are vital to the caterpillar. To the bird it means absolutely nothing whether it is sitting in an oak, a linden, or a birch tree. But for the caterpillar there is a world of difference between one species of tree and another, for the leaves of one it considers a delicacy, while it would starve to death rather than eat as much as one leaf of another.

This example illustrates that the outside worlds of two forms of life can be fundamentally different even in the same environment. The idea of this subjective outside world, first formulated by Jakob von Uexküll, does away with the notion that man is the measure of all things. A bee does not look at the world from a human point of view. In reality, there are as many outside worlds as there are forms of life; bees, dogs, tapeworms, fleas—each contemplates the real world with its own senses and gathers from it whatever is significant for its own existence.

The higher the evolutionary level of a form of life, the richer is its outside world. We must remember, however, that the simpler, more rudimentary organisms are just as well suited to their way of life as the higher forms are to their own. Every animal is adapted to its own natural environment—the amoeba to the slime of a stagnant pond, the hairy ape to the primeval jungle. As long as we regard the preservation of life as the chief goal, each creature is "perfect" in its own fashion. But the higher and the lower forms of life are still separated by an immeasurable gap, the real magnitude of which only becomes apparent when we consider the differences between their outside worlds.

The outside world of the lowest forms of life is inexpressibly bleak. Creatures up to the evolutionary level of the worms hear no sounds and see no colors; many of them live in eternal darkness. Even a human who is blind and deaf has a much more vivid sensory life than these creatures, whose sense of touch and whose chemical sense are incomparably less keen than ours. When the same sense is present in different forms of life, it often functions in completely different ways. A snail, a bee, and a bird, looking at the same object, will all see it differently.

The outside world—the world perceived by the senses—is the source of all that a form of life is and does, thinks and feels. The environment can, however, affect the organism without stimulating the senses. When you stretch out on the beach to get a suntan, you are actually seeking the effect of ultraviolet radiation that cannot be perceived by the senses. The ultraviolet rays penetrate your skin, causing the formation of pigments, and may even give you a painful burn; although these rays are no part of your sensory world, they have a very powerful effect on your body. Even the action of heat is for the most part beyond the range of our senses. Although we notice heat and cold, we are unaware of their real effect, which reaches to every cell in our bodies and influences our metabolism.

Within the world that is available to the senses, however, sensory perception has a clearly defined and profound purpose. It enables the organism to meet actively the forces which operate in its world. No matter how great is the variety of responses with which an organism meets its world, we shall be safe in saying that all those responses are beneficial to the organism. This is the very foundation of the existence of every living creature.

A completely new sensory stimulus disturbs the body's state of equilibrium, and the body reacts by creating a new equilibrium to meet the changed situation. A simple example will show how this works. If you suddenly move from a dimly lit room into the sunshine, the intense light has a disturbing effect. Your eyes react at once:

your pupils contract to cut down the amount of light that enters them. Your reaction to the stimulus thus cancels out, to some degree, the state of affairs that produced the stimulus. Physiologists call this phenomenon regulation; it occurs over and over, in many different ways, in our daily lives. The situation will be more involved at times, but it always occurs as a closed cycle. When hunger sets in, the animal becomes restless. Like a hunter sending out his dogs to track down game, the hungry organism sends out its senses to detect fresh nourishment. When its senses have led it to food, it eats, and gone is the hunger that triggered the whole process. The state of equilibrium that existed before hunger set in has been recovered.

The senses are the reliable guides that lead the organism along the often quite intricate paths of life. But if we wish to understand thoroughly the nature and the action of the senses, we must take a closer look at the whole subject. Our first query will be: What elements of our bodies enable us to receive the stimuli of the outside world?

2. *The Sensory Cell*

To learn how our senses function we must take a close lock at the parts of the body that do the work. Some of these—our eyes, ears, nose—are only too easy to find. Others cannot be seen without a microscope.

The entire human body is composed of cells. In every sense organ are found special sensory cells, each of which is connected with a minute, delicate nerve fiber. When a stimulus excites the sensory cell, the nerve fiber forwards the excitation to the brain or to some other part of the nervous system. (We should note here an important exception. Neither our sense of touch nor our heat sense makes use of sensory cells. Stimuli of this sort are received directly by the nerve fiber itself, which splits up into many delicate branches under the skin. But this special case will be discussed later.)

Before going any further we should probably say exactly what a stimulus is, but unfortunately there is no clear-cut answer to this question. We can say definitely that every stimulus registered by our sense organs is either of a physical or of a chemical nature. This means that as a result of the stimulus a sensory cell either gains or loses energy. In other words, our sensory cells are very sober, very precise workers, some of them physicists, others chemists by profession. In the last analysis even the most soulful glance is nothing but an optical signal, and the most solemn handshake simply disturbs certain of the touch-sensitive elements of one's skin.

The exact process that takes place when a sensory cell is stimulated is still a mystery. The cell sensitive to light —actually a miniature chemical laboratory—has been the subject of the closest study so far. The commonly held view is that when light strikes the cell it causes a substance (which we shall call S) to break down into two components (call them P and A). In the absence of light, these two components tend to combine and form S once more. Thus when the light is strong, the amount of S is reduced, and P and A are increased; in a dim light the situation is reversed. A sustained, uniform illumination produces a state of balance, which is upset as soon as the light changes. Even in a sustained light, however, chemical changes of this kind take place constantly in the visual cells; these changes act as stimuli.

The light that has excited the light-sensitive cell of the eye does not go any farther. It does not enter the optic nerves, and the physical brain is shrouded in darkness even when the sun is brightest. The excitation which the nerve sends from the sensory cell to the brain no longer has anything to do with light. This becomes obvious when we consider how our sense of heat works. When a cold-sensitive nerve ending in the skin is excited by contact with a cold object, it cannot possibly transmit the excitation to the brain as an actual state of coldness. The nerve, which on its way into the interior of the body is surrounded by warm muscles and blood vessels, would obviously lose its coldness to the surrounding tissues.

Specific disposition

Our sensory cells are detectors; they inform the organism of the physical or chemical changes that take place in the outside world. Each of these detector cells is a specialist, reacting only to certain stimuli. A cell sensitive to light cannot be aroused to activity by any sound or mechanical pressure, but it will react instantly to the slightest change in the intensity of the light. A tactile corpuscle, outpost of our sense of touch, will not react to light, and it is just as indifferent to chemical stimuli of any kind. This important property of the sensory cell, its absolute indifference to all stimuli not designed expressly for it, is called its specific disposition; the stimulus to which the sensory cell will react is called the adequate stimulus.

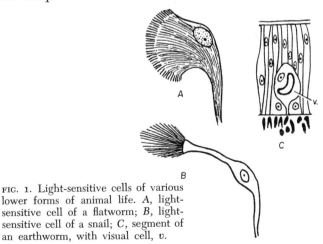

FIG. 1. Light-sensitive cells of various lower forms of animal life. A, light-sensitive cell of a flatworm; B, light-sensitive cell of a snail; C, segment of an earthworm, with visual cell, v.

How this limitation of the sensory cell develops is still a great mystery. The microscope reveals few differences between individual sensory cells, and some of them we simply do not understand. The light-sensitive cells of the lower forms of life frequently have a fringe of infinitely fine cilia (Fig. 1), or contain a remarkable body, the phaosoma, which has a peculiar striation on its edge; but we do not yet know what purpose these developments serve. The other sensory cells likewise fail to display any clear connection between their structure and their function. Only by indirect means can we gain any information about how they work. A chemical cell that registers external stimuli cannot lie deep inside the body; it must extend to the surface of the skin, and such cells frequently show a minute appendage protruding to the outside. It is often very difficult to distinguish them from the tactile cells, for the latter also have such appendages (Fig. 2).

As in most biologic laws, there are numerous exceptions to the law of specific disposition. Time and again some sensory cell will react to stimuli not designed for it. For instance, if you touch a finger quickly and lightly to the tip of your tongue, you will have a distinct sensation of a sourish taste. This observation should not be construed to mean that the human finger has a slightly sour taste, for if you sterilize a piece of platinum wire over a flame, let it cool, and then touch it lightly to the tip of your tongue, you will be aware of exactly the same taste sensation. This experiment proves that the sour taste is a mere sensory illusion, produced by the light touch on the tip of your tongue.

Similar observations have been made on animals. The hind rim of the foot of the mud snail (a member of the family Nassaidae) is equipped with chemically excitable sensory cells. These cells have a definite duty: they protect the snail from its most dangerous enemy, the starfish, by reacting to the exhalation of the skin of that

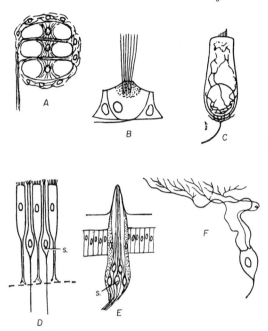

FIG. 2. Mechanical and chemical sensory endings. *A,* tactile corpuscles from the beak of a bird; *B,* a sensory cell from the statocyst of a mussel; *C,* auditory cell of a mouse; *D,* olfactory cells of a mammal; *E,* olfactory cells of an insect; *F,* cutaneous sensory cell of a dragonfly; *s.,* sensory cell.

marine marauder. But the same sensory cells react also to lyes, acids, heat, and electric stimuli. In other words, they are far from being truly selective; in all likelihood the mud snail is never exposed in its natural habitat to these false, "inadequate" stimuli, so that only the "adequate" ones trigger the cells to action.

The conclusion that our sensory cells are chemical or physical devices has advanced our knowledge considerably, but new difficulties loom before us. We have seen that the nerve that links the sensory cell with the brain does not transmit the stimulus in its original form, as

heat, or light, or taste. The nerve is an indifferent conductor, like a telephone wire. It is excited by the sensory
cell and sends the excitation, essentially an electrical
phenomenon, to the brain. This excitation reveals nothing about the nature of the stimulus that has triggered it.
In these circumstances, one cannot help wondering how
the brain learns anything at all of what goes on in the
outside world.

For a better understanding of the situation, think of
how the telephone works. The original stimulus is completely changed between the transmitter and the receiver.
The telephone wire conducts rapidly changing electrical
impulses which show no kinship with the human voice
that speaks into the apparatus. In the receiver, however,
the electrical impulses are transformed into a close re-
production of the voice that acted as the original stimulus. Of course the human brain does not have a receiving
mechanism of exactly this sort, but both processes use a
transmitter, an indifferent conductor, and a receiver. We
must now ask how the brain performs the difficult task
of acting as a receiver.

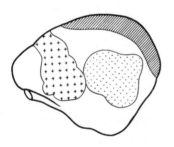

FIG. 3. Sensory projection areas
of the brain of a cat. //// visual
center. ::: auditory center.
+++ tactile center. (After
Woolsey and Fairman.)

The specific energy of the sensory centers

A definite part of the brain is assigned to each sense
organ—eyes, ears, nose, and so on (Fig. 3). The optic
nerve, for instance, runs to the visual center, the *area
striata*, situated in the rearmost part of the cerebrum.

Each of these centers can respond in only one way to excitations from the sensory nerves. Any stimulus will result in the specific sensation characteristic of the center stimulated. For instance, no matter how the visual center is excited the result will be a sensation of light.

This characteristic of the sensory centers is called their specific energy. This term was coined by Johannes Müller, physiologist, anatomist, zoologist, and universal genius. Although the word "energy" has acquired an altogether different meaning in physics and technology since Müller's time, his original term has been retained out of deference to tradition. In combination with the specific disposition of the sensory organs, the specific energy of the centers forms the basis of our entire sensory life.

The sensory cells themselves are not even necessary to generate the specific sensation in one of these centers. Anything that produces a certain change in the nerves leading to the sensory center will evoke that sensation. Nerves react to all sorts of stimuli—to electric currents, to mechanical impacts, and so on. Any manipulation of the optic nerve produces the sensation of optical phenomena. This fact was known even to that famous old teller of tall tales, the good Baron von Münchhausen. Once, while on a hunting trip—so goes his tale—he found himself face to face with a ferocious bear; to his dismay, he discovered that he had lost his flint and had no way to fire his old-fashioned musket. The resourceful Baron, however, punched himself in the eye so hard that sparks flew from it, the sparks ignited the powder in the musket, the shot rang out, and the formidable beast fell dead.

Our pain sense supplies perhaps one of the best-known examples of this sort. After the amputation of an arm or a leg, the patient will frequently feel a pain and insist that he feels it in the limb that is no longer there.

Such a direct excitation of the sensory nerves seldom occurs under ordinary circumstances. In everyday life a sensory center of the brain only experiences an excitation as the result of the excitation of the sensory cells which are welded by connective nerves into an inseparable unit with it. The specific disposition of the sensory cells and the specific energy of the sensory centers work in concert here; the visual center is activated only when light impinges on the eyes, and the auditory center only when sound vibrations excite the ears. This finding, however, does not imply any logical connection between the external stimulus and the sensation within the recipient. There is just no such thing. The sensation "red" has nothing to do with light of a wave length of 800 millimicrons; the odor of camphor and its chemical composition are two different worlds, for which there exists no common point of contact.

The sign language of the senses

Hermann von Helmholtz, the great student of nature to whom we are indebted for so many discoveries in the fields of physiology and physics, was the first man to formulate the principle, based on these facts, that our sense organs do not convey to us a true image, but only signs or symbols, of the world that surrounds us. Our senses are incapable of grasping the true properties of things. We are trapped in the escape-proof prison of our brain and sensory centers. In the light of what we know, this doctrine is no longer a hypothesis, but an indisputable fact. But the human mind rebels against it. Are the solid, tangible things that we behold in this world mere illusions?

In this difficult situation, it is helpful to remember that we employ such signs and symbols time and again in other phases of our lives. Speech, the most intimate of all mediators among human beings, dates back to the very earliest beginnings of human civilization. For countless thousands of years, speech was the only means of communication, as well as the only means by which the wealth of man's experience and learning could be handed down through the generations. Writing was the result of a later, gradual development. But even our writing consists of symbols. The letter *O* has no more similarity to the spoken sound *O* that it represents than that sound has to the sound wave that strikes our ears. A letter is a symbol of a sound, precisely as the sound is a symbol of the sound vibrations, and yet we know very well that conventional written letters or symbols furnish a complete substitute for the spoken word.

Although there is no similarity between the spoken word and the written word, both observe the same order of the elements that make up the word. This is also true of the signs or symbols conveyed to us by our senses. Our eyes and ears reproduce a great many separate details which blend, in the object, in a certain order or sequence. In visual images, this order is of a spatial nature. An experiment will demonstrate this in a remarkable way. The retina of the eye contains a red substance which turns pale when light impinges on it. If you make a vertebrate animal look at a window, then turn off the light and immediately kill the animal, removing its eye and treating the eye with certain chemical reagents, you will see a picture of the window on the retina (Fig. 4). The order of auditory sensations is chronological. Since we perceive sounds in the sequence in which the sound waves reach our ears, the relationship between the physical process that seems as a stimulus and the resulting sensation proves to be much closer than one might have thought.

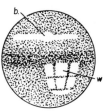

FIG. 4. Optogram of the eye of a rabbit. *b.*, blind spot; *w.*, image of a window.

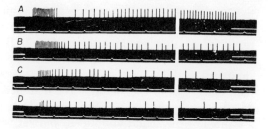

FIG. 5. Action potentials of a single optic nerve fiber of a king crab. Intensity of stimulus: *A*, 0.1 unit; *B*, 0.01 unit; *C*, 0.001 unit; *D*, 0.0001 unit. (After Hartline, 1932.)

3. *The Intensity of the Stimulus*

It is a common experience that the intensity of our sensations increases with the intensity of the external stimulus. But science had to expend a vast amount of effort to find out how this relationship is maintained. The difficulty is not in the sensory cell. Obviously, a light-sensitive cell will react more energetically to a strong light than to a feeble one. But the behavior of the nerve is puzzling because, as we know, it obeys a law of "all or nothing at all." A rifle cartridge obeys the same law. You can "excite" a cartridge by pounding at its sensitive spot, the primer. If you do so, the result will be one of two possible alternatives: you either pound too lightly, in which case nothing happens, or strongly enough, in which case the cartridge will go off. But you will accomplish nothing by pounding away at it harder than is necessary. The cartridge can go off either completely or not at all; there is no such thing as "more" or "less" for it.

If the same law applies to the sensory nerve, it is difficult to explain the dependence of our sensation on the intensity of the stimulus. But we can carry our analogy a little further by replacing the rifle with a machine gun. Although its cartridges obey the law of "all or nothing at all," the machine gun can change the rate at which the cartridges are fired. It took the modern electrophysiological method, which taught us how to record the minute electric currents present in the nerve—the action currents—to clear things up at last. Today we know that the more the sensory cell is stimulated, the higher is the frequency of the electric discharges of the nerve. The higher the frequency, the stronger are the sensations in the brain (Fig. 5).

This discovery has still not told us all there is to know. Everyone has noticed that the sharpness of our vision depends on the brightness of the illumination. If you study a printed poster in the waiting room of a railroad station or in some other brightly lit public place, you can stand a certain distance away from the poster and still can make out the letters and figures on it. If the light is dimmer, you must stand much closer. To explain this fact it has been suggested that the individual visual cells which are our means of viewing the poster have different stimulus thresholds. The meaning of this theory can be made clear by the following analogy. Ten boy scouts fall sound asleep in a cabin after a strenuous hike. What will happen when they are awakened the next morning? One or two of the boys are light sleepers, and even the sound of the footsteps of the man coming to wake them may be enough to rouse them from their slumber; but the others will not wake up until the man begins to pound on the door, and two of them must even be literally dragged out of the bunks before they are really awake. Each of the ten boys represents one visual cell of the human eye; each has his own "threshold." In bright light, each of the visual cells in the compact pattern of your retina is stimulated, and consequently you are able to distinguish a great many fine details. In light of normal intensity, a number of your visual cells will remain inactive because their thresholds of stimulus are not reached; the image is now lacking in fine details—your vision is poorer. Finally, in very dim light your vision is limited to the major features of the object (Fig. 6). This hypothesis is frequently disputed nowadays, but it still remains the most plausible theory.

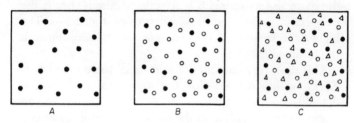

FIG. 6. The dependence of the sharpness of vision on the intensity of the illumination. These drawings are based on the assumption that the individual visual cells have different threshold values. *A,* feeble light—only a few visual cells are excited; *B,* normal illumination; *C,* strong light.

4. The Response to the Sensory Stimulus

Although man's responses to the stimulation of his sense organs are extraordinarily varied, they all fall under one of the following heads: sensation, reflex, or excitation. Let us study this in a little more detail.

The sensations

A person's sensations stand at the innermost portal of his soul and lead into a realm to which nobody but he himself can have access. The sensory world of every being, even of those closest to him, is sealed to him more impregnably than the treasure house of some legendary king, guarded and watched by a thousand armed soldiers. Just what a sensation actually is, nobody can reveal to others; it is a basic phenomenon of life, mysterious as life itself, one that cannot be traced back and reduced to anything else. Many philosophers have taught that our sensations are the only realities, and that we deduce our entire idea of the world from them. Everything in the world becomes known to us through our sensations alone. Without sensations, you could live to a ripe old age without knowing any more than you did in the moment of your birth.

At the outset, in studying this problem, we face a very important question. What about the sensations of other living beings—all the other members of the human race, our domestic animals, as well as the lower forms of life?

Our best course will be to consider humans first. Surely no one will deny that other people are capable of sensations, although we can only judge the sensations of others from our own. Things are no longer quite so simple when we consider animals, even animals of the highest orders; for all practical purposes we must conclude that we cannot make any statement about the sensations of animals. This does not mean that they do not exist, but simply that our knowledge reaches a barrier that we cannot cross. To claim that because we cannot perceive sensations in animals these sensations do not exist would be like saying there is no dark side of the moon because we cannot see it. In a human being, a sensation is frequently the only effect produced by a stimulus. Visual, aural, and tactile stimuli often produce no reaction at all. When we do react to an optical or acoustic stimulus this process always takes place indirectly, through the mediation of the preceding sensation. First we see, and this act of seeing brings about the decision to reach for the object seen, or to undertake some other action.

Reflex movements

The predominance of sensations is likely to lead to the misconception that a sensation is the only way of reacting to sensory stimuli. It is easy, however, to see that this is not true. The organism will in innumerable instances react to a stimulus by a movement. Such a movement may be accompanied by a sensation, but there are also cases where a reflex movement occurs without the accompaniment of sensation. Everybody knows that the pupil of the eye reacts with machine-like precision to every change in the light that falls on it. But unless you hold a mirror in your hand you will not notice this reaction, because the contraction of your iris is not accompanied by any sensation.

The reflex movement of the pupil is another method, equal in importance to sensation, of reacting to certain stimuli. A reflex runs its course along a definite nerve path (Fig. 7). The excitation is conveyed from the sensory cell to the sensory center, exactly as in the case of a sensation; from the center the excitation is forwarded,

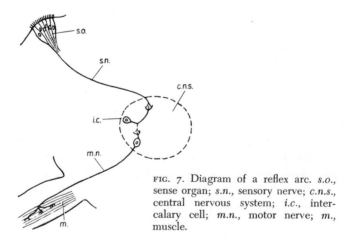

FIG. 7. Diagram of a reflex arc. *s.o.*, sense organ; *s.n.*, sensory nerve; *c.n.s.*, central nervous system; *i.c.*, intercalary cell; *m.n.*, motor nerve; *m.*, muscle.

usually by way of relay stations, to a motor nerve which conducts it to the muscle concerned. Just as your doorbell begins to rings when somebody presses the button outside, the muscle linked to the reflex arc jerks with machine-like accuracy whenever sensory cells connected with it are stimulated.

The reflex action of the pupil of the eye is one of the simplest reflexes known to us. It is completely independent of our control. The mechanism is more complicated in other cases, but reflexes play a far more important part in our lives than is ordinarily surmised. Many of our "voluntary" movements are voluntary only in the beginning; we trigger a complicated reflex mechanism which then runs its course automatically. The movements of the eyes provide a good example. Most people are completely ignorant of the fact that they have six ocular muscles, and even if they did know it, they would still be unable to contract any single one of those muscles deliberately so as to make their glance fall on any desired object. As you form a decision to look at an object, you trigger a reflex mechanism which starts from your retina, runs its course in a most complicated fashion over the midbrain, and ends at the ocular muscles. In this and in similar cases, you are doing no more than the driver of an automobile when he shifts from first to second gear—with a simple movement of his hand he activates a mechanism whose operation may be a complete mystery to him.

It may seem that volition comes out on the short end, but this is not so. The organism that reacts to a sensory stimulus is no slave to its senses, no reflex-action robot. The organism makes use of its reflexes as its most lowly servants, although without these servants it would be totally helpless. In the hierarchy of our central nervous system—a far more involved and intricate one than our bureaucratic systems—the reflexes are usually organized in a certain pattern. A primary reflex center, similar to that associated with the pupillary reflex, is subject to an inhibitory center, which ordinarily impedes the execution of the reflex movement. This inhibitory center, finally, is controlled on the highest level by still another center which cancels out the effect of the inhibitory center whenever the organism so desires. In this way the unruly reflexes are pressed into the service of the organism.

The excitation of the nervous system

The third function of the sense organs—the excitation of the nervous system—is just as important as sensations and reflex movements. Everyone is familiar with the ancient story of mighty Samson who lost his strength when Delilah cut off his hair. Science has revived this old legend, but in its version the hair is replaced by certain sense organs. One of these sense organs is the labyrinth, the intricate organ that includes both the apparatus of equilibrium and the organ of hearing. In all vertebrates the labyrinth is served by the eighth cranial nerve. Figure 8 shows a pigeon whose labyrinths have been removed. A small ball of lead is tied to its beak; the bird would ordinarily be able to carry this small weight (about ¾ oz.) without difficulty, but it is now so weak that the ball pulls its head down. The working of the labyrinth is an oddity; its sensory cells constantly send excitations to the nervous system, even when no external stimulus acts on them. There are many examples of the importance of such organs. The powerful common crab, whose claw can ordinarily crush a pencil with the greatest of ease, becomes a pitiful weakling upon removal of its organs of equilibrium, the statocysts.

Muscular strength, which is based on impulses of the nervous system, is not the only characteristic dependent on the sensory apparatus; so also is the motility of the body. If the spinal cord of a shark is severed from its brain by an incision and the fish is suspended in an aquarium, uniform wavelike movements will ripple over

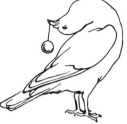

FIG. 8. Pigeon with labyrinths removed. A small weight is attached to its beak. (After Ewald.)

the slender body for hours and hours. These movements are the product of the constant motor impulses sent by the spinal cord to the body. But these impulses are by no means "spontaneous." If the experimenter severs all the sensory paths running from the sense endings to the spinal cord, the fish remains motionless. The impulses which the spinal cord, when intact, keeps radiating to the muscles are based ultimately on the excitations which reach the spinal cord from the skin and from other parts of the body.

The most convincing proof known to us in this domain concerns the lower forms of life. The rocky shores of the Mediterranean are the habitat of a shy marine worm, the *Hydroides uncinatus* (Fig. 9). Its entire body is hidden safely in a calcareous tube, and only its delicate head

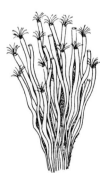

FIG. 9. Part of a colony of *Hydroides uncinatus*.

with its plumelike crown of pinnae protrudes. Whenever
the light changes a little, whether dimming or brighten-
ing, the worm retreats with the speed of lightning into
the safety of its tiny fort. One of these creatures will
ordinarily respond to an increase of a few per cent in the
brightness of the light. But if you leave one of them in a
totally dark room for a few hours, and then suddenly
turn on a strong light, not a single fiber of its body will
react to this extraordinary stimulus with as much as a
twitch. The darkness has made it unable to react even
to the most powerful illumination. If you leave it in the
light again for a while, its sensitivity to light will slowly
return.

We learn a similar lesson from the small, lively medusae which dart about in the sea in the spring. Many of
them, the so-called Anthomedusae, have four small,
flame-red eyes on the rim of protruding bells. The purpose of these organs was unknown for a long time, but
an experiment has given a surprising answer. The medusae keep making spasmodic swimming movements,
without which they would sink down to the bottom of
the sea. Physiologists call them "swimming hearts." If
you put the creatures in a glass bowl and keep the bowl
in a dark chamber for a few hours, one creature after
another will cease its swimming movements, and finally
all of them will lie on the bottom. When brought into
the light they begin making their swimming motions
again, and soon all the medusae are swimming about
merrily. This experiment demonstrates that the small red
eyes do not serve as organs of sight, as one would be
likely to surmise, but that their chief purpose is to excite
the nervous system so that it will make the muscles
twitch.

Scientists for a long time paid no attention to these
phenomena; nothing analogous had ever been cbserved
in human beings—for the simple reason that the mechanism of the human body is far too complicated. A

es

sensory cells from the hidden depths of
ntact and undamaged, we might be able
hey respond also to pressure and other
uli. Within the ear, however, each of
only to sounds of a quite definite pitch.
ory cell cannot react to pressure or other
uli for the simple reason that, hidden in
he skull, it is never exposed to any such
pecialization of these cells is likewise easy
nd is conducted first of all to a vibrating
hich consists of approximately 20,000 tiny
ely side by side. A sound will produce a
ibration only in that fiber which is in
h it, and this vibration is transmitted only
cells linked with the particular fiber. Thus
he ear's ability to distinguish various sounds
narily on the mechanical structure of the
on the specific nature of different "auditory

gan and the central nervous system

f their close link with the external world, our
create the outside world that is the basis of
life. It would be wrong, however, to con-
the entire intellectual development of the
gdom is the consequence of the increase in
cy of the sense organs. An equal importance
cribed to the efficiency of the central nervous
remarkable agency which receives and proc-
timuli registered by the sensory endings and
by the nerves. In our survey of the evolution of
ense we found a great range between the scat-
-sensitive cells at one end of the scale and the
structure of the human eye at the other; we
onfront the lowest with the highest when we
he nervous system of a coelenterate with the in-
e seat of the soul of man, his brain.

modern experiment, however, brought final conviction. We have learned how to register the minute "action currents" which indicate the state of the excitation of each individual part of an animal's nervous system. If you bring two fine electrodes in contact with the nervous system of a river crab, you will find that the electric discharges become much stronger when one of the crab's eyes is exposed to light. This is a direct, firsthand demonstration of the stimulating effect of exposure to light. Of particular interest is the fact that this effect will persist for a considerable time after the light is extinguished and the eye is in darkness again.

Sensation, reflex movement, and excitation of the nervous system are thus the three different effects which the sensory stimulus is capable of producing. They frequently run parallel but independent courses, without interfering with each other. They are like three very dissimilar sisters; each is of the highest importance in its own fashion, but the supremacy must still be conceded to sensation, which represents the foundation of our entire life.

5. *The Sense Organs*

Individual sensory cells are not found scattered over the skin; in most cases a great many of them are combined in a higher unit known as a sense organ. In every form of animal life, and in every sensory domain, the same pattern occurs: a group of sensory cells is surrounded by an apparatus whose task is to increase the efficiency of the sensory cells. The astounding degree of development that is possible becomes evident when we compare the human eye with that of a snail, or the human ear with an insect's.

How does this development actually take place? The best example is provided by the sense of light. Organs sensitive to light form a continuous series ranging from the simplest eyespots to the most highly evolved, compound, lens-type eyes. The eyespot of a medusa, for instance, is more efficient than the light-sensitive skin areas of other forms of animal life, because in the medusa the sensory cells are clustered much more densely together. Such an organ may be regarded as an amplifier. This statement applies to practically every existing sense organ.

Still more significant is the fact that a more highly developed sense organ generally permits the organism to make finer distinctions—to perceive more than it could with a mere group of sensory cells. In the visual sense, the first improvement occurs when the visual cells are recessed instead of being situated externally on the skin. Many sea snails and marine insects have such eyes (Fig. 10, *B* and *C*). With such an eye the organism can discern the direction from which the rays of the sun are coming; this knowledge helps the creature move about. The next evolutionary jump is a big one. The "pit eye" closes almost completely, except for a small hole, where the light rays can enter; the organ becomes a true optical apparatus, a sort of rudimentary box camera (Fig. 10, *D*). When the light is strong enough, this "camera" can project an inverted image of the environment onto the retina. This odd apparatus is found in the oldest cephalopod still existing, the *Nautilus*.

As the next step on the evolutionary ladder, the "pit eye" closes completely, becoming a fully enclosed eye which, as a rule, shows an important optical improvement: a lens. Our land snails have such eyes, and they are also occasionally found in animals of a very low order, for instance in certain Chaetopoda and certain medusae. As is demonstrated by cameras and by the human eye, a lens can greatly improve the production of the image; but in these very primitive cases the lens probably only serves as a condenser. In a box camera without a lens, only a very narrow pencil of rays radi-

FIG. 10.
organ of
simple eye
pound or
(See text.)

ating from a so
equivalent. As a
allows the eye a
rays that reach i
point on the retin
sent a much brigh

Only in two gr
the vertebrates (F
higher and make us
lary action and close
create mechanisms
production of image
evolution justifies the
nism of the sense org
the richer is the out
ganism.

Such auxiliary device
senses. In all likelihoo
auditory cell in the tru

remove the fine
the human ear,
to prove that t
mechanical sti
them will react
Why? The sens
mechanical sti
the maze of t
stimulus. The
to explain. So
membrane, w
fibers set clos
sympathetic
resonance wit
to the sensory
we find that t
is based pri
ear, and not
cells."

The sense o

Because o
sense organ
our mental
clude that
animal kin
the efficien
must be as
system, th
esses the
conveyed
the light s
tered ligh
miraculou
likewise
compare
explorabl

Let us take a little closer look at the relations between the two agencies, the sense organs and the nervous system.

Among the innumerable forms of animal life that thrive in the warmer oceans are the remarkable Cubomedusae, so named for the rectangular cross-section of their bodies. Naturalists are interested chiefly in their extraordinarily developed eyes. These eyes are seated on the marginal bodies, pedunculated organs hidden in considerable numbers in small pits on the margin of the bell (Fig. 11). Each marginal body has several such eyes, which are not simple pigment spots but look quite like the eyes of small vertebrates. We can distinguish a

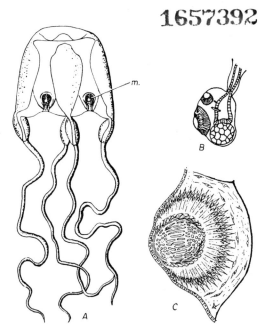

FIG. 11. The Cubomedusa *Charybdaea marsupialis.* A, the animal as a whole; B, marginal body with eyes and statocyst; C, magnified cross-section of an eye; *m.,* marginal body.

big, spherical lens, a vitreous body, and a well-developed retina in the background. What is a medusa doing with such an intricate eye? This eye should be able to produce some sort of image, but this ability would be totally useless because in place of a brain the medusa has only an irregular aggregation of nerve cells at the base of the marginal body. No one has yet succeeded in discovering the true function of these eyes, but it seems likely that they gather the dim light that reaches them and, like so many magnifying glasses, increase its stimulatory effect by concentrating it.

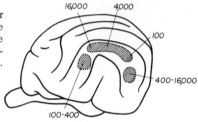

FIG. 12. Auditory center of the brain of a dog. The figures indicate the wave lengths of the sounds perceived in different areas.

From this first example we deduce that there are two fundamental requisites for the seeing of an image. First, there must be an eye capable of registering an image, and second, there must be a brain capable of interpreting and comprehending that image. The first element, the eye, is useless if the second one, the brain, is missing. Only in the highest forms of life has nature achieved something like perfection in combining the actions of sensory apparatus and nervous system; for this reason the intricate problem has been studied mostly in mammals. The method of recording facts by electrical devices has led to some amazing discoveries. If you attach electrodes to the brain of an anesthetized animal and then stimulate a certain sense organ—for instance, the ear—certain of

the electrodes will register an electrical discharge, showing that that part of the brain is linked with the organ in
question. A systematic exploration has shown, for instance, that the lateral fields of the brain of the dog
include a region where the receiving apparatuses for a
great many sounds are lined up side by side in an orderly
sequence according to pitch (Fig. 12). The "receiving
stations" designed for the highest sounds occupy the
immediate foreground, while those attuned to the deep-
est sounds are situated in the rear. Beside them there are
two more compact areas, one of which processes only
the deep sounds, the other all the higher ones. In the
preceding sentence I used the word, "processes," as a
hint that we know nothing more definite about them.
All we can say is that this is where the electrical excitations of the nerves are transformed into sensations.

The system is much the same in the other senses. In
general, for each peripheral "transmitting station" there
is a "receiving station" in the brain (Fig. 3). It is amazing
to see how these relationships develop with the increasing evolutionary level of the organism and its specializa-
tion in certain sensory domains. The sense of touch, for
instance, is represented in the brain of a rabbit by a small
spot in the temporal region. The snout of a pig is extremely sensitive to touch, but the rest of its body is
rough and insensitive; apparently, the snout is the only
part that is represented in the brain by a sizable area.
Dogs and cats use their forepaws in many ways, especially for capturing their prey and for eating, and the
sense of touch of these limbs is well represented in their
brains. The same limbs are represented to a far lesser
extent in the brains of the hoofed animals, which use
their legs solely for walking and standing. In the brain of
the primate there is a long, narrow strip which relates to
the entire body. The largest area of this strip is linked
with the face and the arms, but the back, the hind legs,
and even the tail are also represented.

The area linked with the sense of sight lies in the rearmost zone of the brain. This area is of course much more developed in the human brain than in the brain of any other animal. The human brain has not only a general visual center, the *area striata*, but also a special area reserved for optical sensory images, and furthermore an optical speech center, situated slightly on the side. Experiments cannot be performed on living human subjects, but the pathologists have supplied us with an inexhaustible store of material. When a patient suffering from a visual disturbance dies, a post-mortem examination can reveal exactly what part of his brain failed to function properly.

Consideration of the co-ordinated action of sense organ and brain may lead us to philosophical speculation. A comparison of a lower animal, such as a codfish, with another animal of identical size but of a higher order, such as a cat, reveals (Fig. 13) that the sense organs of the codfish have outstripped its brain in their development. The eyes of a medium-sized codfish are quite similar to the eyes of a cat in their size and internal structure. If sight depended on the eyes alone, the codfish would be able to see and distinguish as well as the cat. Experience teaches, however, that the fish is a rather stupid creature, with a limited ability to make rational use of its eyes. It snaps at whatever it sees; if the prey happens to be too big for it to tackle, the codfish knows enough to seek safety in flight. It can recognize its female, as well as its rival for her affections, and the two males will fight it out. But this is about the limit of the natural abilities of a codfish. In planned experiments, it can, of course, be trained to perform all sorts of tricks. It will learn to recognize various letters of the alphabet, and can be taught to swim to certain letters and to avoid others. But it requires human guidance and assistance for such accomplishments.

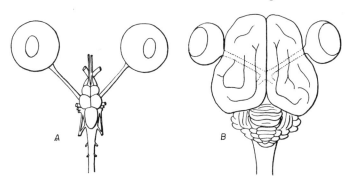

FIG. 13. Eyes and brain of, *A*, a codfish, and *B*, a cat, reduced on the same scale. (Original.)

To understand why a fish sees so much less than a mammal of the same size, we need merely compare their brains (Fig. 13). The fish cannot make full use of its eyes because its brain is too poorly developed. This statement may be in general applicable to every form of animal life. Probably no living creature can use fully the stimulations received through its sense organs. Most of what an animal perceives through its senses rebounds from the impenetrable wall of its intellectual inadequacy.

The peculiar lag of the brain behind the sense organs is, however, the ultimate motive of the ever-increasing intellectual development in the animal kingdom. Whenever the brain adjusts its performance ever so slightly to meet the demands of the sense organs, the outside world of the organism immediately expands; if conditions are favorable, the way is open for the organism to take a step forward on the evolutionary scale. This is not just a a theory of some armchair scientist. If you will but scan the history of our world, you will find that the prehistoric animals were infinitely more stupid than those living today. The brain of every one of the mighty saurians of the Jurassic era was so small that it was a most difficult task for the scientists to locate the space it occupied in the skull of the animal.

Life on our planet is unquestionably still evolving. We may well shudder to think of what huge heads our descendants will have in the next geological era!

6. *The Site of the Senses*

We human beings, accustomed to regarding ourselves as the measure of all things, are inclined to take it for granted that every animal carries its most vital sense organs in its head. Man sees, hears, smells, and tastes with his head, and only what are referred to as "lower" senses—those senses which have not evolved enough to form true sense organs—are scattered over other areas of his body. Animals often show a very different picture. The sense organs which are intended to inform the organism about the outside world are always located where they can best receive the stimuli, and that location may vary greatly according to the way the animal is built. In most animals the head occupies a privileged position, but it has no monopoly. As a matter of fact, what *is* a head? The simplest multicellular animals known to us, the sponges and the Hydrozoa, have nothing of the kind (Fig. 14). They are radially symmetrical, very much like flowers, and "front" and "rear," "right" and "left" are meaningless terms with reference to them. In the opinion of the experts, this arrangement of the parts of the body in a circle about a central point is linked with the fact that the creatures are sessile—they spend their lives rooted to one spot, like flowers, or float freely in the ocean. Eons ago, other animals evolved from them; these new evolutionary forms learned to crawl about, and as they adapted themselves to this new way of life they

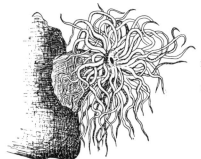

FIG. 14. Sea anemone (*Anemone sulcata*) on a rock.

gave up the radially symmetrical shape. Their bodies divided into right and left halves, and they became accustomed to crawling in a certain direction; thus the function of "forward" came into being. The forward end of the animal was naturally the first to receive the stimuli of the outside world; it was thus the site where in most cases the eyes and the organs of smell and of touch developed. When at last the mouth made its appearance the "head," as we know it, was complete. It is a good general rule that the head is the site of the most important sense organs, but this rule has a number of exceptions; we will now take a look at some of the exceptions.

The mussel once had a head, which has since disappeared. The region where the head must have lain is between the two shells, where no stimulus of the outside world could possibly have reached it. All sense organs have disappeared from this site, and only the mouth and the small brain mark the place. The most important sense organs, the eyes and the olfactory tentacles, have shifted to the outermost part of the mantle by which the shell is formed. Here they are in contact with the outside world.

Eyes appear in all sorts of places. Certain sea snails and the Onchidium, the lazy, light-shy animal found in the sea under rocks, have a number of eyes on their backs. Light striking the broad back acts as an alarm signal for the animal, warning it to creep under a rock to hide. The timid tube worms, which retreat into their shells with lightning speed at the slightest disturbance, often have eyes on the outermost tips of their tentacles. These small eyes act as sentries, like lookouts on a tall watchtower. Among the relatives of this creature is a small worm which has two eyes on the rearmost tip of its body. This worm usually lives in a tube, with only its front end showing, but it can leave the tube whenever it pleases. When the worm goes out in search of a better place to live, its long tentacles, folded together umbrella-fashion, make it difficult for it to crawl forward head-first. As a result the worm has developed the habit of crawling backward; the two eyes on its rear serve it as excellent guides.

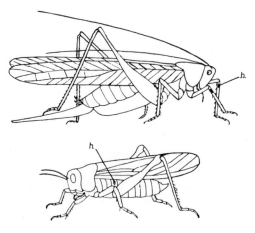

FIG. 15. Site of the organ of hearing, *h.*, of a locust (above) and a grasshopper (below).

It may strike you as funny that grasshoppers and crickets carry their auditory organs on their abdominal surfaces or on their legs (Fig. 15). Of course it really makes no difference where the receptor apparatus is located, because the auditory sensations are always formed in the brain. Two facts may help explain why the auditory organs of these insects occupy such a remarkable site. First, it can be demonstrated that the auditory organs of the insects evolved from other sensory cells that might be formed anywhere on the body or limbs, but never on the head. Second, the head of an insect is in most cases very tiny, providing no room for a tympanic membrane. Strict logic prevails in this arrangement too: it was not by accident that the auditory organs of these creatures developed where they are.

Let us now take a look at the chemical sense. We will discuss later the biological significance of this particular sense; for the time being it is enough to point out that we have both a short-range and a long-range chemical

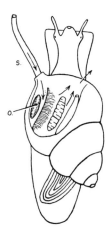

FIG. 16. Gill-breathing snail with olfactory organ (osphradium), *o.*, in the mantle cavity. *s.*, siphon.

sense. The long-range sense enables a form of life to tell its quarry from those other forms of life which it has reason to fear, as well as from other members of its own species; the short-range sense aids the organism in investigating its food. In man, the site of the long-range sense is the nose. As you draw a breath, the stream of inhaled outside air sweeps past the folds of the mucous membranes of your nose. This combination of breathing and smelling is found in other forms of animal life as well; wherever the organ of breathing is located you also find the organ of smell. The gill-breathing aquatic snail, for example, has a long, tubelike organ, the siphon, which extends into the water; the siphon draws in water, which passes through its gills (branchiae) into its respiratory chamber (Fig. 16). Before the water reaches the gills, however, it passes through the peculiar organ of smell, the osphradium, which for this reason is situated not in the head, but in the respiratory space.

Crustaceans have a similar system. Their most important olfactory organs are the first antennae—very small structures situated well in front on the head and bearing the olfactory hairs—in their exposed situation they are eminently suited for their task. If these appendages are removed from a common crab, the crab does not lose its capacity for long-range chemical perception. In these animals, the respiratory water streams from the rear forward. If you place a tiny bit of meat behind a crab, it will reach backward with its claws, between its legs, and seize the meat without turning around. Such experiments made many investigators wonder whether there might not be chemoreceptors (organs capable of receiving chemical stimuli) situated in the respiratory cavity of the crustaceans. Such structures have indeed been found in great numbers in the river crab.

The short-range sense of chemical perception, commonly called the sense of taste, is usually found in the mouth or near it. There are important exceptions; we know, for instance, that the soles of the front feet of many butterflies and flies are extraordinarily sensitive to taste stimuli. This peculiar feature is wholly functional. Flies and butterflies frequently eat overripe fruit fallen from trees—food that is large enough to permit them to walk about on it.

The butterfly is lured to the food by its scent. As the butterfly flits erratically about in the air, it perceives the scent; flying in a constantly narrowing spiral about the tree, it alights on the ground near a fallen piece of fruit. It will then proceed straight to the fruit; as it steps on a spot on the skin of the fruit, where the sweet juice has collected, the gustatory stimuli on the sensory areas of its feet cause the rolled up feeding tube to extend.

7. Pleasure and Displeasure

A sensation is evoked in your mind by everything that you see or hear, by the colors of a bunch of freshly picked flowers as well as by the dismal gray of an autumn day, by the strains of a Beethoven symphony as well as by the ear-splitting caterwauling of cats in your backyard at night. All these sights and sounds produce sensations, but each of them affects your mind in a different way. Pure colors and sounds delight your heart, clashing mixtures of colors or dissonant noises annoy you. Certain stimuli are pleasant, certain ones unpleasant.

The theory of music shows that there is a close link between the purely physical frequency of sound waves and the tonal effect they produce. If a chord is to be pleasing to the ear, the frequencies of its component sounds must bear a simple mathematical ratio to each other. The same principle holds true in the realm of colors: pure, rich colors which contain only light of a certain wave length are the ones most pleasing to the eye.

This remarkable relationship between the physics of stimulus and sensory pleasure has not yet been scientifically explained. We can, however, recognize still another law: the same stimulus can be a source of either pleasure or displeasure, according to the conditions under which it acts. An experience of my own will illustrate this point. In my student days, I happened once to dip my cup too freely in a bowl of delightful strawberry punch, and for the next five or six years I felt the most violent loathing for that particular fruit. My pleasure had suddenly turned into displeasure. Experiences of this kind are frequent, and everybody must have had at least one of them. Such a change is a common occurrence in expectant mothers. Many pregnant women are revolted by the very thought of foods that they normally consider delicious.

Sensory pleasure

Narrow-minded people regard sensory pleasure and the enjoyment of life if not as outright inventions of the devil, at least as incompatible with the serious philosophy of life which rests on the two somber pillars of reason and duty. Those who are closer to the founts of life know that sensory pleasure is an indispensable guide on man's journey through life.

The pleasures derived from eating, for instance, serve a profound purpose. Physiologists once used to judge the value of foods by their calorie contents alone. Each gram of fat, albumin, or carbohydrate that you introduce into your stomach gives you a certain amount of physical energy that can be expressed in units of heat, as so many calories. Your body needs this energy as a steam engine needs the energy supplied by coal. But if your cook served you merely a mixture of these substances, even though they are very important per se, you would be highly indignant. The taste of the food has absolutely nothing to do with these sources of energy; flavor is the product of all sorts of admixtures of other substances that, although they lack all calorie content, perform an important duty in whetting the appetite. Appetite not only makes the eater "dig into his food" more enthusiastically than he could without it, but aids the proper functioning of his intestinal canal.

The smell or sight of a tasty dish makes the saliva gather in one's mouth. This is a useful process; the saliva not only helps your food slide down your throat faster, but contains a ferment that is important in the digestion of all farinaceous substances. The great Russian scientist Ivan Pavlov demonstrated further that the stomach begins to secrete the important gastric juice with added enthusiasm when the food tastes or looks good. This is the famous "appetitive gastric juice," the bridge across the gap between man's sensory pleasure and the processes that take place, unknown to him, deep within. The better a food tastes, the better it is digested, because of the abundant flow of the appetitive gastric juice. This is an example of the physiological effect of sensory pleasure, measurable in conformity with the strictest scientific methods.

When a child refuses to swallow a dose of vile-tasting cod-liver oil, his mother will bribe him with the promise of a piece of chocolate. Although the child knows nothing about vitamins and their beneficial effect, he will swallow the medicine simply to get the delicious bit of chocolate. This is no mystery to anybody, but very few of us realize that our daily lives are a part of the same pattern. Just as a mother guides her unreasoning child by offering him a reward, so does Nature guide us, who regard ourselves as intelligent. A normal person, for instance, eats because he likes the taste of the food and because he is hungry. The fact that the food contains a certain number of calories and vitamins was still completely unknown a mere hundred years ago, but few people starved to death from refusing to eat. We do not act for the sake of the physiological effect; in this respect we are no smarter than the child who swallows the cod-liver oil simply to get the chocolate.

The higher forms of life, and possibly the lower ones as well, would have become extinct a long time ago if it were not for the pleasures of love—which are thus more important than anything that reason is able to produce. As in the case of eating, there is no logical linkage between the sensory stimulus which leads to the act and its result. No animal, not even on the highest evolutionary level, has any inkling of the biological significance of the act of procreation—and human beings often wish that they had none either.

We have spoken almost exclusively, in this connection, of human beings. Have we the right to assume that the behavior of animals is also ruled by sensory pleasure? Many naturalists of the past proposed the rather daring theory that in the animals the reflexes and other automatic nervous functions take care of everything, so that animals have no need at all for pleasure or grief. In the highest animals, such as the dog and the cat, the element of pleasure can be demonstrated beyond doubt. Such an animal, which cannot be denied to have a certain awareness of the scheme of things, strives stubbornly for a sensory stimulus known to it by experience; it would be a strong distortion of the facts to reject pleasure as an explanation. Almost everybody has seen some dog or cat absolutely out of control upon hearing the noise of the meat grinder in the kitchen scratch away at the door until permitted to enter. We can avoid many a false interpretation if we only bear in mind that animals, too, can feel happy.

It is undeniable that some dogs love music. I once observed a dog that would urge its mistress day after day, often at a certain hour, to play music for it. It would give her no rest until she took her small mouth organ from a cabinet and the familiar airs sounded in the room. Then the dog would sit back on its haunches and break out in a howl that simply defies description.

If any of my readers feels inclined to do so, I suggest that he put a package of catnip in front of his cat. The otherwise intelligent animal will at once act as if it had gone absolutely mad. It will behave as if every conceivable earthly delight had been showered on it at once. We regret that the poor human race knows no substance which can produce sensations of a similar nature in a human being. Throughout recorded history man has sought such substances and has almost achieved this goal many times. The cat will first sniff carefully at the package; then, hugging the package tenderly to its body it will roll around on the floor, growing gradually more frantic; finally the cat hurls the package away and races after it around the room. In the end the animal is in a state of absolute ecstasy, the sight of which will convince any spectator that cats can experience pleasure.

As for man, there is usually a drop of gall mixed in his cup of joy. The gods have reserved the gift of total, unconditional surrender to joy for children and for animals, and it does one good to share their enjoyment as a spectator.

Displeasure and pain

While pleasurable sensations are the most powerful motives that make human beings and animals perform biologically important acts, the unpleasurable ones are designed by Nature to deter unreasoning creatures from doing things that could result in harm to them. We are acquainted with a great many such sensations within our sensory world: loathing, pain, and bitter tastes are but a few. Their presence serves a purpose similar to that of pleasant sensations.

The feeling of loathing is brought on in human beings chiefly by certain odors. The smell of putrefaction emitted by a decaying animal carcass and the foul odor of feces indicate clearly that a danger of infection or poisoning makes it advisable to give them a wide berth. We arrive at this conclusion through logic, but in an actual emergency we need not think: we turn away in disgust because the dangerous substance offends our senses. Here again our action is not aimed directly at the goal Nature intends to reach. This is another example of how cleverly Nature makes us do the right thing.

The devious course of Nature is no less obvious in the instance of pain, which in one way holds a special position among our senses. Whereas our other sensory perceptions can be accompanied by sensations of pleasure or displeasure, pain is always unpleasant. A man tormented by an agonizing toothache or by a severe burn may think that pain is an invention of Satan. The physician and the naturalist know better. What would the world be like if there were no such thing as pain? If you happened to lean against a hot stove, you would not be aware of the damage until the smell of burnt clothing or flesh reached your nose.

This is absolutely true, you might argue, but what is the biological importance of a pain in one's appendix? To be sure, it is useful to a modern civilized person; if the pain did not make him aware of his plight, he might never get a chance to call the physician. But what does an aborigine in the jungle, or an animal, gain by being tortured by a pain that he can do nothing about? Despite the validity of this argument, pain has some value even in such a case. It stops the savage from pursuing his normal activities, compelling him to lie down and thus get the same benefit we get from resting in bed during a convalescence. This is by no means a real solution, of course. The Biblical words, "In pain shalt thou bear children," express the bitter truth that pain is the hereditary companion of every human being, without his even knowing why. Pain simply does not seem to know where to stop. But despite its inefficiency pain is in general a strict guardian, a relentless disciplinarian, ever ready to warn us against acts which could injure our bodies.

Should pain be regarded as a universal property of all forms of animal life? The experts disagree considerably on this point. In the opinion of many naturalists it is unreasonable to think of a pain sense in a fish, a fly, or an earthworm. These scientists regard pain as a sensation, and since we are forever barred from finding out anything about the sensations of other organisms, they feel that we cannot reasonably talk about it.

This resignation strikes me as unnecessary. I shall therefore attempt to say something sensible about the pain sense of animals. Let us begin, however, with man, in whom pain is by no means a simple matter of sensation. Imagine that it is a balmy afternoon in late summer. You are seated in your garden, peacefully munching on a piece of pie, when an insolent wasp, which regards your pie as its own legitimate booty, plunges its stinger into your lip. A great many things will happen then. First of all, it is more certain than "death and taxes" that you will stop eating. Moreover, you will emit a powerful bellow, and if the wasp did a particularly good job you will leap from your seat and race wildly about the garden. These are objective criteria of the pain sense that are easy to classify: interruption of the action in progress, shouting, and purposeless expressive movement.

Equipped with these observations, we can now approach the animals. We shall find no difficulty in observing the same manifestations in an organism closely akin to us, such as a dog. I recall vividly the moment when my dachshund Kaspar became so absorbed in hunting down a bothersome flea that he carelessly sat down on a bumblebee. The flea was instantly forgotten, a piercing howl rent the air, and the victim took to his heels, his tail between his legs. The entire complex of manifestations is thus identical in the cases of man and dog, and we can justifiably conclude on the ground of analogy, since we cannot do so by direct deduction, that the dog does indeed have a pain sense.

The lower vertebrates, lizards, frogs, and fishes, present a somewhat different problem. They lack the most important mode of expression: the ability to produce sounds. No matter how horribly such an animal is mistreated, it suffers in silence. But they, too, react with expressive movements. When they experience something that would produce the sensation of pain in a human being, some will kick frantically with their legs, others flap their tails, and still others twist and contort their slender bodies. Some even roll their eyes, like a human being in agony. It does not seem to be too unreasonable to credit these creatures too with the ability to feel pain.

There is not too much that we can say about the invertebrates. So vast are the differences between us and these forms of life that we cannot state with any degree of certainty that a snail or earthworm does or does not possess anything similar to the human pain sense. The single exception is the squid, which also have many other features in common with the higher forms of life. The location of their sensitivity to pain is amazingly similar to the location of man's. As every surgeon knows, man's outer skin, the inner lining of his body cavities, and his pericardium (the thin membrane that surrounds his heart) are highly sensitive to pain. On the other hand, his internal organs and muscles show very little sensitivity. The situation is exactly the same in a squid, except that this animal's reaction to pain (its expressive movement) differs greatly from that of man: if you cut the skin of a squid or touch its delicate peritoneum, it does not cry out, but will discharge the contents of its ink sac. On the other hand, you can perform any operation on its internal organs without eliciting any noticeable reaction.

Insects probably have no pain sense at all; at least there is no proof of it. A striking comparison leads us to this conclusion. If the nerves in a rat's leg are severed so that the leg becomes insensitive, the animal may devour its own paw. A healthy rat, one normally sensitive to pain, would never do that; Nature has provided it with this protection. An insect, however, even a healthy one, may on occasion behave exactly like such an enervated rat. If a flesh-eating caterpillar happens to touch with its mouth a bleeding wound on its own body, it will begin to feed on itself. Such carnivorous caterpillars have, in fact, been noted—not by our old friend Baron von Münchhausen, but by reliable experts—that ate up sizable chunks of themselves. This could not happen if they had anything like a pain sense.

We cannot very well believe the story of Baron von Münchhausen that his horse kept charging forward after a cannon ball had torn away its hind quarters, but bees seem to be really capable of doing something just like that. While a honeybee is busy sipping honey, you can slice off its abdomen without disturbing it in the least.

PART TWO:

The Eight Senses—and the Others

Our grandparents were taught that a man must use his five senses if he would go his way through the world without stumbling. We have become wiser in this respect, for we know now that we need a few more senses than those five. Let us take a brief look at each of our senses.

Of first importance in our perception of the outside world is our sense of sight. Second in rank is our sense of hearing which, although it gives us less information about the outside world, is an indispensable link between an individual and the rest of the human race. The set of five senses includes, moreover, the senses of smell, taste, and touch. It is amazing that the temperature sense, which enables us to perceive heat and cold, was not long ago recognized as a sixth sense; we use it again and again in the daily routine of living. A seventh, entirely independent sense that people failed to recognize as such is the muscular sense, the sense that enables you to judge whether you can manage your suitcase yourself or have to hire a porter to carry it for you. Finally, there is the pain sense, the study of which requires no special education. Thus we reach the conclusion that the old doctrine of five senses is inadequate.

Scientifically speaking, even eight is not the full number of the senses. We shall make the acquaintance of the sense of equilibrium, also called the static sense, which we neglect because it conveys no sensation. We shall find in addition that deep within the human body there are all sorts of other sensory perceptions that have nothing to do with the external world, but are of great importance for the regulation and control of our own body movements.

So much for human beings—but what about animals? Are the many species of animals endowed with senses which, although alien to us, aid each species to perceive its outside world? This question cannot be answered with certainty, for only a small fraction of the animal kingdom has been studied closely from this point of view. But we need not expect any great surprises when we do find out. Generally speaking, the senses of all animals—deep-sea, land, and winged creatures alike—are attuned to the same natural stimuli. We may claim with confidence that no animal has, for instance, a sense organ that enables it to perceive electricity or magnetism directly. When we discover faculties which exceed our own, they are instances of a higher evolution of one sense or another, never something wholly new. To be sure, the vision of a bird is eight times keener than ours, the sense of smell of a dog is utterly baffling to us, and there are many animals that perceive sounds beyond the auditory range of the human ear—but in all likelihood we shall not come across anything new anywhere.

We may therefore confidently use man's senses as our guide in the study we are going to make.

1. Sight

Our outside world is composed of the diverse impressions that reach us from the sensory realms. If we stop to consider the share each sense has in the formation of this world, we realize that the eye is the sense organ to which we owe the most. As you sit alone in your room your other senses will be only mildly active; street sounds, ordinary smells and tastes, the touch of your clothing and of the chair you are sitting in reach your senses. But your eyes will make you aware of a thousand and one things—the cabinets full of miscellaneous objects, the books on the shelves, the pictures on the wall— and each of these things will speak to you in its own language and be ready to tell you its story. Whatever you do, the impressions supplied by the sense of vision are rarely overshadowed by those from the other senses.

Our eyes supply our minds with such a wealth of data about the outside world because the impressions conveyed by the eyes are mostly long-range ones. The principal function of all our other senses is to inform us of what goes on in our immediate environment. This is all that our temperature sense, our sense of touch, and our sense of taste can do. It is a rare exception when we catch the scent of trees in blossom or the odor of a chemical manufacturing plant from a great distance; and as for our sense of hearing, the main thing is, after all, to understand the words of the people near us.

Shape perception

In your earliest infancy, when you still viewed everything about you with wonder, a great deal of what you saw registered as empty forms. Gradually thereafter you became acquainted with the meaning and practical uses of a thousand things, and the older you grew the richer this knowledge became. One crams everything that one knows about a thing into the image of that thing. Whenever you perceive the image, you recall everything that you have learned about that particular object. In other words, multiple associations have formed between the optical image and the other sensory impressions generated by the same object. This characteristic does not depend on any particular sense. Your nose and ears also convey many such associations to you. But sight is by far the most important, because a person has a thousand times more opportunities to associate things with what he sees than with what he smells, hears, or perceives by his sense of touch. It is clear that our eyes are foremost among the tools with which we construct and mould our outside world.

This ability of our eyes is called shape perception. What role does this ability play in the lives of creatures other than man? In former days, people naively took it for granted that the eyes of all other forms of life functioned exactly like our own. The difference was believed to be merely that some animals could see better and others less well than a human being. We shall find, however, that the eyes of an insect or of a snail work in an entirely different way, one that is totally alien to us; and that only our nearest relatives, the other vertebrates, are endowed with a shape perception similar to our own.

The faculty of shape perception is indicated by the ability to recognize a familiar object by sight alone, without using the other senses. This faculty can be recognized in dogs, cats, parrots—in short, in mammals and in birds. A dog can recognize its master through a glass window. A crane will recognize its owner in any garb— in formal wear, in a business suit, in beach attire. Even a fish, a creature so very low on the scale of intellectual development, can be taught to react to shapes. As I mentioned before, fishes can distinguish the letter *L* from the letter *R*—definite proof of their faculty of shape perception.

On the other hand, in the invertebrates—insects, spiders, crayfish, and worms—the faculty of shape perception is, generally speaking, so poorly developed as to be hardly worth considering. Appetizing as a fresh leaf of lettuce looks to a hungry snail, if the animal is separated from it by a sheet of glass so that it cannot smell it, it will not take the slightest notice of it. Nor will a love-smitten male butterfly pay any attention to his lady if she is enclosed in a glass cage, even though she is in full view. It was believed for a long time that the bees were

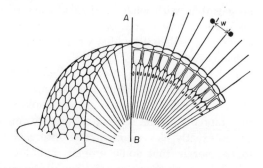

FIG. 17. Faceted eye of an insect. The drawing shows two mutually perpendicular cross-sections running through the axis *AB*. On the right, the individual visual organs are intersected centrally. *w.*, the width of the ocular facet. (After Hesse-Doflein, modified.)

a special case, in view of their amazing accomplishments in other areas of sensory life, but even they have proved dismal failures in this respect. It is an absolute waste of time and effort to try to train a bee to react to a certain shape, such as a triangle, a square, or a pentagon. The best that can be said for the bee is that by natural instinct, without training by man, it prefers intricate shapes to simple ones.

The only invertebrates that may be credited with a certain faculty of shape perception are the large-eyed squids and the graceful jumping spiders. These spiders must be able to perceive shapes, for the males perform a regular mating dance in front of the females; without mutual recognition, this behavior would be inconceivable.

A microscopic study of the eye of a lower animal shows why these creatures have such a poor sense of shape perception. Helmholtz once said that if any mechanic ever dared deliver to him an optical instrument that was as bad as the human eye, he would throw the man out on his ear. Well, the eyes of an insect or a snail are a thousand times worse. This difference can be measured accurately. Make two dots two-fifths of an inch apart on a piece of paper. A human being with normal vision can distinguish these dots at a distance of several yards. Now a bee, like all insects, has compound eyes— the eye is composed of many facets, each of which constitutes a unit and sees only one single white, black, or multicolored blotch. In order for the bee to see them as distinct entities, the two dots must be separated from each other by a distance not less than the width of such an ocular facet (Fig. 17). Each facet covers an angle of approximately one degree. Thus if two dots are two-fifths of an inch from each other, a bee cannot see them as separate dots from a distance of more than three inches.

As we move on to the other lower forms of animal life, eyes become even worse. Whereas the eye of a bee contains several thousand facets, the eyes of snails, spiders, worms, and most of the smaller insects are equipped with only a few hundred (Fig. 18). Their entire field of vision can therefore consist, at best, of a few hundred blotches. That is poor equipment, and so it is understandable that these creatures have been doing without shape perception altogether.

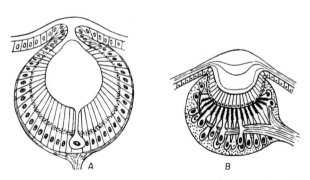

FIG. 18. Lens-type eye of *A*, a chaetopod, and *B*, a spider, showing the small number of visual cells. (After Bütschli.)

Motion perception

It must be admitted, however, that shape perception is probably not very important to most of these creatures. Nature has endowed them with a much simpler and yet almost infallible means of finding their bearings in their world. For them anything that moves is alive, and must be watched because it may be a foe or it may be something to eat; anything that does not move is lifeless and not a source of danger. For two vast groups of animals, the hunter and the hunted, there is all the difference in the world between a creature that sits motionless and one that runs, crawls, or swims about. The motionless being is simply ignored; to be sure, the retina registers its shape, but the brain, the watchful guard, takes no notice of this image. But no sooner does the image of a body in motion flit across the retina than there is a deluge of reports of this significant event, and the brain is instantly ready to take the necessary measures (Fig. 19).

For countless animals, the perception of movement in the outside world plays the decisive role in catching their prey. A tree frog will pay no attention to a motionless fly, nor a salamander to a worm at rest, but their wide-opened mouths are ready at the first sign of movement. The shape of the prey is of no importance whatever. Such animals can, as a result, be easily tricked, and this is, essentially, the secret of the art of fishing. There is just one more thing that interests the animal: the size of the thing that moves. The principle that governs the behavior of such an animal is simple enough in this respect, too: "If it is smaller than you, attack it; you might tangle with something your own size, but you had better flee when you meet up with something bigger than you, or else you may wind up as its meal."

The perception of motion is also useful to many animals when mating. To the senses of a male housefly the

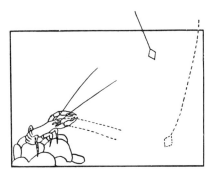

FIG. 19. Motion perception of a crusta-
cean. The animal follows the seen object
with its long antennae. (After Doflein.)

female of its own species is a small black thing flying
through the air. This trait makes it easy to snare male
houseflies. All you need is a long thread with a sticky
black ball the size of a housefly fastened to one end of
it. Pull the thread through the air at a moderate speed,
and soon some love-hungry male housefly will be trapped.
Females, on the other hand, can never be caught in this
way.

For a familiar demonstration of this type of vision,
think of the shying of a horse. The wild horse, in its
natural habitat, is a fleet-footed dweller of the plains,
and the stealthily stalking predatory beasts are its natural enemies. To be able to escape them, the horse has
eyes that do not see straight ahead, as ours do, but side-
ways. While the horse is feeding, it can see a great many
things that take place to the side and almost behind it.
To be sure, a horse cannot perceive sharp images with
those parts of its retina that serve this purpose, but that
is not the important point. Anything that moves—a piece
of paper, or a shirt on a clothesline fluttering in the wind,
or a car speeding by—triggers off a sharp reaction. To
see and to flee is the matter of a split second. True, the
horse shies more often than is necessary, but rather a
hundred flights too many than one too few!

The way in which movement-oriented vision aids in the detection of an approaching enemy is demonstrated by the scallops (Fig. 20). Scallops rest on the bottom of the sea, but they are much more alert creatures than their sluggish relatives, the common edible mussels and the oysters, which live only to eat and to digest. The many small, glittering eyes of the scallop, circling the edge of its mantle, keep a lookout for the approach of an enemy —in particular the starfish. A starfish may look quite harmless at first glance, because it has neither claws nor teeth and crawls along so slowly, but once a creature is

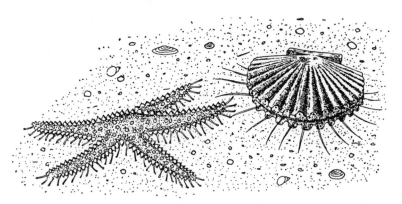

FIG. 20. Starfish and scallop equipped with olfactory tentacles and eyes on the mantle edge.

caught in the murderous embrace of the innumerable sucker-disks on its feet, there is no escape. The scallop is always on guard. As the image of a slowly advancing larger body moves across the retinas of its many eyes, the retinas alert a second line of sentry posts. The big tentacles situated between the eyes extend an incredible length toward the advancing enemy. If they recognize the scent of the death-dealing starfish, the scallop takes flight at once, swimming by clapping the two sides of its shell together.

Photo-orientation

The majority of the lower forms of life rely on light that comes directly from the sun. Creatures on a higher evolutionary level, whose eyes are better developed, can react to light reflected by other bodies in their environment. This ability is possessed both by organisms whose vision is oriented toward motion and those whose vision is oriented toward shape perception.

Directional vision is something so unusual to us that we must accustom ourselves to the very idea. In everyday life it is totally unimportant to us from what direction the rays of the sun are coming. Even in the desert, where it is easy to lose one's bearings, the position of the sun is not all-important if one carries a compass. The Chinese are said to have invented the compass before the birth of Christ, but it was never used in Europe until the twelfth century. How, then, did the ancient Greeks and Romans find their way on the high seas and in unknown lands?

A very interesting answer to this question appears in Xenophon's *Anabasis*. When Xenophon led his Greek troops from what is now Turkey to Greece, he wanted to head for the Black Sea to the north. Breaking camp at dawn, Xenophon tells us that he marched "with the sun to the right." In other words, he used the sun exactly as we use a compass today. In both cases, if the marcher keeps a constant angle between the direction of the march and a constant point of reference, he knows that he is moving along a straight course.

Insects that spend a major part of their lives on the move—the dung beetle, the ground beetle, the ant, the running spider, the bee on the wing—all use the same principle Xenophon used 2500 years ago. The sun is their

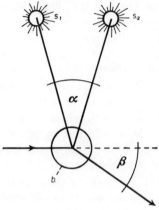

FIG. 21. Photo-orientation. *b.*, dark box; *s.*₁ and *s.*₂, positions of the sun; $\alpha = \beta$. (Brun's experiment.)

guide and compass. An ingenious method will show that this is true of ants. The experimenter finds an ant that is hurrying on its way. Casting a shadow over the ant, he uses a mirror to make the rays of the sun reach its eyes from the opposite direction. The result is striking: the insect stands still for an instant, then makes an abrupt about-face, pivoting on the rear of its body, and scurries back, retracing its steps along the route by which it came. There is an even neater experiment. An ant that is headed for its nest is captured and kept in a dark box for an hour or so; when it is released from the box, it does not continue along its old route, but chooses a new one that deviates from the former by the same angle by which the position of the sun has shifted in the meantime (Fig. 21).

This behavior, which can be designated as photo-orientation (orientation by light), has disclosed an important secret of the world of these small creatures. But a further question arises at once: Why do these tiny wanderers in the great world need to go in such a straight line? To be sure, the ant represents a different case because it wants to get home to its nest, but the ground beetle and its kind have no home; the whole world is their hunting ground! We need not ponder long over this particular problem. The German poet Goethe, unacquainted as he was with photo-orientation, found the perfect answer with the inspired vision of the true seer. In *Faust*, Mephistopheles says:

> In all his search for knowledge, prideful man
> Is like a beast that wanders round and round
> Misled by fiends through dry and barren ground
> While all about are fields of pasture green.

Translated into terms a beetle would understand, this poetic statement means: "If you do not find food where you are, you will surely starve to death if you keep running around in a circle. You must move forward, in a straight line, if you want to find something to eat." Every small creature follows this directive with unerring instinct.

A beetle marching in a certain direction relative to the sun can very easily lose its bearings. Say it falls into a wheel rut and crawls laboriously up the steep bank of dirt. When it regains the road, it is immediately aware that its position is all wrong; the sun now shines into its left eye, whereas before its mishap the sun was on its right. No matter what position the beetle is in, it can always regain its former direction relative to the source of light.

Let us assume that a dung beetle, which was originally following a course such that the sunlight met its left eye at right angles to the longitudinal axis of its body, now stands so that its right eye receives the light at an acute angle from a point in front of it; in this situation, the odds are ten to one that the insect will turn clockwise. In other words, it will turn through the lesser angle (about 135 degrees of arc) to resume its original position relative to the light. On the other hand, if in its new position the light shines into its right eye at an angle from behind, the beetle can be expected with a great degree of certainty to turn counterclockwise (Fig. 22).

Phototaxis

Photo-orientation is not the only known form of directional vision. A man lying sick in bed, spending endless hours in weary brooding, or one idly musing while he waits in the anteroom of some big shot, may realize suddenly that his eyes are fixed on the bright ceiling light, as though under some magical compulsion. This phenomenon seems to be a vestigial remnant of primitive habit, still found among the lower forms of animal life, which is known as phototaxis or phototropism.

The effect of phototaxis is such that as soon as the animal becomes aware of a source of light—the sun, the

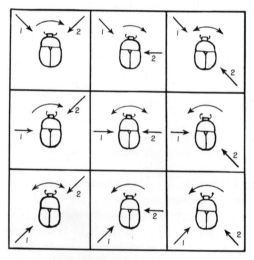

FIG. 22. Reaction of a dung beetle to a change in the direction of the light. Light *1* is replaced by light *2*. The arrow indicates the direction of movement by which the beetle re-establishes its original position relative to the light.

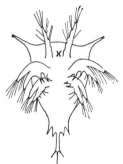

FIG. 23. Larva, in a later nauplius stage, of a barnacle.

sky, or an electric bulb—it immediately turns in that direction and hurries toward the light, usually in a straight line. Phototaxis may also manifest itself as an aversion to light: the animal may flee the light, running, swimming, or flying in the opposite direction.

What is the meaning of this strange behavior? It is certain, first of all, that no animal regards the source of light as a desirable object in itself. All animals are earthbound creatures; flying to the sun would do them no more good than it is said to have done Icarus, who fell into the ocean when his waxen wings melted in the sun. The light is merely a road sign which beckons phototactic animals to itself. No further general statement can be made about phototaxis; a study of each specific instance can reveal how the form of life involved benefits by following the light. Let us discuss a few specific examples.

Barnacles are small crustaceans, members of the genus *Balanus,* that live in the sea, firmly attached to rocks, wharf piles, or even to the shells or bodies of other marine animals. In the spring, shortly after the mating season, the protective shell of a barnacle harbors a host of its tiny offspring, the nauplius larvae, ready to emerge into the great world. These larvae are tiny creatures with six strong, bristly legs (Fig. 23). Cyclops-like, each has a single eye at the foremost point of its head.

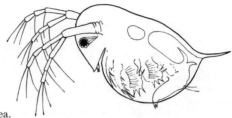

FIG. 24. Water flea.

As soon as the nauplius larvae have left the protection of the maternal shell, an irresistible urge propels them toward the light. The direction of the light is not quite the same under water as it is on land, for sunlight can penetrate the water only at a steep angle. In the evening and in the morning, the slanting rays of the sun cannot pierce the water because its surface acts as a reflector. Whatever light there is under the surface of the water almost always comes from straight overhead. The small barnacle larvae, as well as countless other creatures— worm larvae, clams, snails—swim up from the bottom, seeking the light. Once they near the surface, they are scattered in all directions by the current and the waves, so that the offspring of a single mother are soon dispersed over a wide area. When they have had their fill of swimming toward the light, they sink to the bottom and seek a quiet place, where they attach themselves firmly for the rest of their lives. In this instance, phototaxis is the agency that prevents all the offspring of one mother from settling in her immediate vicinity, where they would eventually be compelled to engage in ruthless competition with each other.

Since laymen will probably never get a chance to observe such occurrences directly, I shall describe an experiment by which anyone can produce phototaxis. The only apparatus required consists of a large glass vessel and a siphon bottle filled with carbonated water; the experimental animals will be a handful of water fleas

(*Daphnia pulex*), the tiny crustaceans you can buy in any pet shop (Fig. 24). In warm weather, vast crowds of water fleas bustle about in lakes and streams, and everyone has seen them there. But their love of the light is not apparent under normal circumstances. If you put a few thousand water fleas into a jar full of water, let them swim about for a while as they please, and then squirt some carbonated water in the midst of that carefree crowd, you will witness a sudden change. Every single water flea seems to be possessed by the desire to reach the light; they swim in dense swarms toward the transparent glass and keep butting their heads against it.

It is easy to prove that the carbonic acid in the charged water squirted among them makes the water fleas become positively phototactic. Phototaxis in this case is the result of an interesting interaction among different senses. The carbonic acid is a chemical stimulus; it is perceived by the chemical sense organs and reported to the brain. As this report is registered, a change takes place in the nervous system. The visual apparatus, which heretofore has served other purposes, is readjusted to phototaxis, and the effect is evident at once. In the glass vessel, the behavior of the water fleas is totally meaningless. They die eventually, poisoned by the carbonic acid, no matter how hard they batter against their glass prison.

The meaning of this complicated process becomes evident only as you visualize how it occurs in nature. The bottom of a pool where the water fleas live is a scene of decay; animal carcasses lie there decomposing, and leaves blown into the water by the wind sink down and rot. All this rotting organic matter generates a vast quantity of carbonic acid, which poisons the water. The water fleas must flee such danger spots. Since light always enters the water from overhead, phototaxis is a simple aid to their flight: it guides them away from the poisoned water at the bottom to the surface where the water is safe.

We can study phototaxis in many familiar forms of animal life right in our homes. By doing so, we may even learn something useful. For instance, nobody likes the fat green bottle-flies that love to invade your bedroom through an unscreened window early in the morning. If you use phototaxis, you can chase them out in a matter of seconds. Just take a towel or some other large object and chase the flies about the room. When they become frightened, phototaxis sets in, and they head straight for the bright window and safety.

These three examples will enable you to form a somewhat more concrete idea of how phototaxis works. In each of these cases, it rescues the animal from a situation of distress and leads it to a more congenial place. The life of the animal may be in danger, it may be threatened by poisoning, by asphyxiation, or by violence. Seeking the light is an automatic reaction the significance of which they do not understand. Nature uses the light to guide these tiny creatures safely away from danger.

The cutaneous light sense

Strange as directional vision seems to us, it is nevertheless something that we can duplicate with our own eyes. But the cutaneous light sense, the scientific term for which is photodermatism—the ability of an organism to use part or all of its outer skin as a light-perceptive organ—is fundamentally inconceivable to us. Yet a great many animals, in the most diverse zoological classes, have no other way to perceive light. Instead of eyes, these creatures have light-sensitive cells scattered over the expanse of their skin, just as spots sensitive to heat or to pain are scattered over the human skin. Such an animal is incapable of sight in the sense in which we customarily use this word. If light waves produce any sensation at all in these creatures, they probably perceive them as we perceive heat.

The cutaneous light sense unquestionably produces reflex movements, the most complicated of which is the movement toward or away from light; this movement obviously comes under the heading of phototaxis. The mechanism can be illustrated by analogy with the human heat sense. No human being would have any difficulty locating a hot stove or the entrance to a cold cellar in total darkness. As you approach the door of the cellar, you feel cold air against, say, your right hand and right cheek, while your left hand and cheek register nothing of the sort. You need only turn until you feel the cold air strike your face from straight ahead, and you will know that the cellar entrance is directly in front of you. This is exactly how a light-shy earthworm manages to avoid brightness. When the light strikes it, it turns until the light shines on its body directly from the rear, and then it can reach the comfortable darkness by crawling straight forward.

An eyeless animal is capable of such light-oriented movement only if its body, like our own, can be divided into a left half and a right half, so that it notices whether the two halves are equally or unequally illuminated. Most forms of animal life meet this requirement, but the majority of the single-celled beings are completely asymmetrical. Many of them are nevertheless capable of finding their way into the darkness—among these is the well-known ciliate *Stentor*. The method employed by a stentor is simplicity itself. Whenever, as the animal swims aimlessly about, its particularly sensitive front end reaches the borderline between light and shadow, it recoils quickly as if it received a shock, then turns a little, changing direction, and sets out once again. This process of trial and error may be repeated three or more times until the animal remains in the shade as it swims on.

The cutaneous light sense serves not only to locate the environment where the degree of light best suits the organism, it can also protect the animal from danger. A certain aquatic worm lives in a calcareous tube that protects its delicate body, but its little head with its fine crown of tentacles protrudes into the water, exposed to any and every attack. This creature must be constantly on its guard, or else some voracious fish might suddenly swoop down and bite off its head, tentacles and all. If the worm had eyes its job would be easy, but its only warning devices are its cutaneous light sense and the high sensitivity of its tentacles to vibrations. These two properties must protect it. If a fish approaches from the dark side, the tiny creature will become aware of it by the movement of the water; if the marauder comes from the bright side, its shadow will cause the worm to retreat hurriedly into its tube.

A shadow is an important alarm signal to many such eyeless creatures. If a shadow appears all of a sudden, it cannot be cast by a cloud passing overhead. If it falls on a large expanse of skin or a great many tentacles at the same time, it cannot be cast by a small animal. It must signal the approach of some creature of respectable size, and therefore, danger. Of course there are a great many peaceable fishes that harbor no evil intention, but since this worm is unable to recognize its real enemies it must avcid every potential danger. This simple philosophy of life governs the behavior of a great many of the lower forms. Each of them carries it out in its own fashion. If a shadow falls on a clam, it immediately snaps its shell shut; a snail will pull in its horns and a gnat larva that was just about to rise to the surface of the water for some fresh air will wiggle back into the depths. On the other hand, the sudden increase of a thousand candle power in the light will not make the slightest impression on these creatures. No increase in the degree of brightness can mean anything exciting in their lives.

If you stroll on the beach at low tide and observe the sand at your feet, you will notice many remarkable forma-

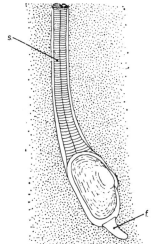

FIG. 25. Sand clam, *mya arenaria*.
f., foot; *s.*, siphons.

tions like the figure eight. Each of these consists of two black holes linked by a short bridge—the top view of the tube which is the home of the white soft-shell or sand clam, *Mya arenaria*. Figure 25 shows a cross-section of the animal and its home. You can see the foot that dug the deep hole, then the shell, and above it, extending into the water, the pair of siphons—two long hollow tubes whose open ends fill the figure eight. One of the siphons keeps sipping up water, and along with it the thousands of minute algae and other delicacies the clam eats; the other siphon ejects the used water.

The siphons are fleshy, tasty morsels for any predatory fish. If they extended unprotected into the water, the clam would soon be minus these important parts. But the clam's cutaneous light sense protects it from such a disaster. As soon as the light-sensitive tips of the siphons are touched by the light of day, they give an alarm signal to the nervous system; in a matter of seconds the appendages are withdrawn into the protection of the sand.

2. The Color Sense

The importance of the color sense among the human senses is demonstrated eloquently by the interest which the very greatest intellects have devoted to this question. Leonardo da Vinci, Newton, Goethe, Helmholtz, and many others, including great men of our day, have made valuable contributions to chromatology, the science of colors. Yet not one of these great thinkers has really succeeded in clearing up the mystery of the color sense, and it will probably be some time before mankind attains any satisfactory understanding of it. For this reason, the following paragraphs are not intended to be a learned discourse on our present knowledge, but simply a few general remarks about the color sense.

A comparison of sound and light may prove to be enlightening. In nature there are thousands of sources of sound—the animals, the wind, the murmuring brooks, footsteps, thunder, the surge of the surf, and so on—but only one source of light: the sun. The auditory sense of an animal is often tuned to one specific source of sound, but the color sense of all living creatures is adjusted uniformly to the properties of sunlight.

If we ask a physicist about the sunlight, he will tell us that it is composed of many rays which differ from each other only in their wave lengths. There are no colors in physics; colors exist only where there are organisms that see colors. A blend of all the rays of sunlight seen together looks colorless—that is, white—to us. The colors we see thus owe their existence not so much to the sun as to a most peculiar fact. Most of the objects about us absorb certain light rays and reflect others. A poppy looks red because it absorbs the yellow, the green, the blue, and the violet rays and reflects the red ones right into the eyes of the spectator.

Although we are all familiar with these experiences, their explanation is far from simple. Physics and chemistry are still unable to give any satisfactory explanation of color. That sulfur is yellow, that cinnabar is red, and that coal is black are simply facts that one has learned, as one has learned the date of some important event in history. This peculiar behavior of objects with respect to the rays of the sun is, however, quite useful to us. If an organism knows how to distinguish light of different wave lengths, it has acquired an extensive new ability: it can distinguish between objects that reflect different colors.

The significance of the color sense becomes most obvious when we think of the colors we find in nature. In our asphalt and concrete modern cities natural colors mean little, but in nature color still plays its important role. Chlorophyll enables the foliage, which needs solar energy, to take the best possible advantage of the rays of the sun. Flowers, which made their appearance in a much later era, needed to be seen; they therefore dressed in brilliant hues that would stand out against the green foliage—blues, yellows, red, white. Their splendor did not spring into being for our sake, but to please the bees, the butterflies, and the other busy insects that fertilize the flowers. The flowers and the insects, which constitute one of the most intimate symbiotic systems known to men, grew and developed more or less together. For this reason the color sense of the insects, with its simplicity and biological clarity, is best suited to serve as an introduction to the entire subject.

The color sense of insects

Let us begin with the butterflies. You will find that it is very easy to study the color sense of these graceful creatures. A butterfly that has just emerged from the cocoon contemplates a new world with its new senses. Put a number of bright red, yellow, green, blue, and violet paper flowers on a gray background before the butterfly and then simply count how many times it visits each flower. The butterfly does not need to learn anything; when it leaves the cocoon every ability, every knowledge that it will need for its simple, brief life comes along with it, ready-made. A liking for bright colors is one of those congenital traits.

From the moment when the butterfly's wings have hardened so that it can fly, a flower is a powerful magnet to it. A tabulation of its landings on the brightly colored paper flowers yields a remarkable picture (Fig. 26). Most of its flights end on the yellow and the blue paper flowers; it visits the red, yellowish green, and violet ones very sparingly, the green ones practically not at all. Of course, such observations do not warrant the conclusion that blue and yellow are the only colors a butterfly can see; they merely demonstrate its color preferences. But tastes differ even among butterflies. The *Vanessa poly-*

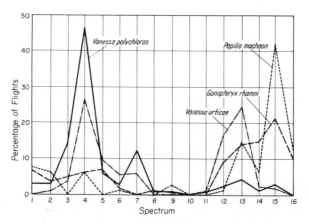

FIG. 26. Tabulation of the results of an experiment designed to test the spontaneous color preference of different butterflies. On the spectrum, 1–3, red; 4–5, yellow; 6–7, yellowish green; 8–9, green; 10–11, bluish green; 12–13, blue; 14, violet; 15–16, purple. (After Ilse.)

chlorus wants to feast only on the honey of yellow flowers, the *Papilio machaon* prefers violet ones. All these tiny creatures are naturally conditioned, as it were, to certain colors. Green, not at all popular in these tests, is a favorite of the female of the cabbage butterfly (*Pieris rapae*) when she prepares to lay her eggs.

In order to learn more about the color sense of insects, one must train some of the little creatures to respond to different colors. Bees have proved to be particularly valuable subjects in these studies. They teach us that the insect eye does not perceive the full range of colors that reaches the eyes of human beings. When there is a rainbow in the sky, the bees see only four color bands. The first of these extends from our bright red to our green, the second consists solely of the narrow strip of bluish green, and the third one comprises our blue and violet. But the four comes to the layman as a big surprise; the bees see as a distinct color something to which the human eye is totally blind: ultraviolet radiation. On the other hand, the bees are unable to see red, which appears black to them.

Reflect on the practical consequences of such a primitive color sense. Visualize, for instance, a bowl containing a bright red apple, an orange, a lemon, and a bunch of green grapes. To our eyes, each of these fruits is differently colored, but a bee would see all of them as being of the same color, although some would be lighter and others darker. Perhaps even more striking is that to a bee all the yellow flowers—goldenrods, buttercups, sunflowers, and so on—differ from the background of green foliage and grass only in brightness, but not in color.

What color is a poppy? A human being will declare that the poppy is red, because he cannot see ultraviolet; a bee, which cannot see red, sees the poppy as ultraviolet. The difference in the vision of the two can be demonstrated by an ingenious experiment. If you cover the poppy with a transparent glass bowl, through which no ultraviolet radiation can pass, the bee will pay no attention to it. If you replace the transparent glass bowl by one made of black glass, which is penetrable only to the ultraviolet radiation, the poppy will become invisible to human eyes, but bees will fly straight to it.

The limited range of the insect's color sense has had a profound effect on the development of our flora. Practically none of our flowers is a solid red, because a solid red flower would look black to most insects. On the other hand, many flowers that look rather drab to human eyes—for instance, the bryony, *Bryonia alba*—contain an ultraviolet color component, the splendor of which is inconceivable to a human being.

The color sense of vertebrates

We must not make the mistake of assuming that only the mammals have a good color sense, and that other vertebrates do not. Many mammals roam about in the dark of the night and sleep through the bright day in some dark hiding place; they are often equipped with a very limited color sense or with none at all. No animal below the level of the primates seems to have a truly good color sense comparable to ours, although a passably well-developed color sense is present in the hoofed mammals as well as in the domestic cat. In fact even the very lowliest members of the vertebrate clan, the fish, can distinguish as well as can man the colors of the rainbow in its many-hued splendor. A fish can therefore be trained to respond to orange, or to yellowish green, or to bluish violet. It will never confuse one of these colors with its immediate neighbors in the spectrum.

It must be admitted, nonetheless, that only the study of the human being will improve our knowledge of the color sense. It soon becomes evident that a study of objective movements for which animals are the only available subjects will not suffice; we must use a subject who

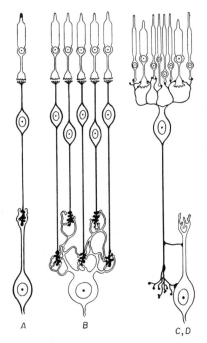

FIG. 27. Details of the retinas of primates. A, cone, traced in isolation; B, 5 cones, traced as a large ganglion cell; C and D, various rods and cones, traced jointly. (After Polyak, 1941.)

A   B   C, D

can report on his own sensations. Our next step, hesitant as it will be, will take us into the maze of the human color sense. Our survey will be limited to the fundamental facts.

Rods and cones

The retina of a vertebrate differs from the retina of any other living creature in that it contains two different sensory cells, rods and cones (Fig. 27). These two types of visual cells have different functions. The cones are for day vision; they enable us to see in bright light, and we also owe to them our ability to see colors. The rods, on the other hand, are active when the light is dim, chiefly at night; we cannot distinguish colors with them but only shades of brightness.

These visual elements are distributed in the human retina in a special way. In the center of the retina, in the *fovea centralis* (the pit in the middle of the so-called yellow spot) there are only cones, and no rods at all. From there toward the periphery of the retina the number of cones decreases and the rods become more and more numerous. The *fovea centralis* is of paramount importance in our vision. This tiny spot is the only place where you see a sharp image. If you see something in the lateral field of your retina and want to investigate it more thoroughly, you turn your eye so as to cause the image of that object to be projected exactly onto your *fovea centralis.*

There is a very simple way of demonstrating that there are no rods at all in the *fovea centralis.* On a clear night, when you are looking at the starry skies overhead, try to look closely at a fixed star of medium magnitude. The result is surprising. When you bring the image of the star onto the *fovea centralis,* as you are accustomed to doing when looking at things in the daytime, all that bright splendor will suddenly be gone, because that spot is devoid of rods. If you glance a little to the side, the star will just as suddenly reappear.

The rods give rise to all sorts of questions. As the full moon "fills hill and dale with silver sheen," all colors are blotted out in that radiance. The fairy-tale silvery glow swallows up both the green of the vegetation and the bright riot of colors of a flowery meadow. I do not know whether it was this sight that induced Goethe to conclude that the moon emitted a light different from that of the sun. He was wrong, of course. The moon borrows its light from the sun, and the only difference between moonlight and sunlight is a difference in intensity. Sunlight is approximately 160,000 times as strong as moonlight. We ourselves create the silver hue of the moonlight by looking at it with our color-blind rods.

From our knowledge of man we conclude that the

retinas of all nocturnal creatures—toads, mice, rats, bats, and what have you—are equipped with rods only. On the other hand, there are many diurnal animals, especially among the reptiles, whose retinas have only cones. Such animals will see colors even by moonlight, but will in all likelihood be unable to make out anything as soon as it becomes dark.

The three-color theory of vision

In every sensory act there are two elements: one is the sense organ, which reports to us what is going on in the world around us, and the other is the brain, which translates the signals of the sense organs into sensations. These two agencies, through which all sensory impressions must pass, are as different from each other as they can possibly be; but if you test your sense organs by self-observation, you will be unable in most instances to determine what effect is to be ascribed to one and what effect to the other of these two agencies. The scientists of earlier eras found it impossible to get over these difficulties, and only in more recent times were methods worked out to permit the function of the sense organ to be distinguished clearly. Some inspired students of nature nevertheless anticipated a great many years ago what practical experiments did not succeed in proving until quite recently.

The earliest, and therefore perhaps the most important, of these men was the English naturalist Thomas Young (c. 1800). He knew nothing of rods and cones or of the sensory cell, for the cell theory was not even formulated until half a century later. But Young had an inspired idea: that in order to distinguish the different colors, the eye must contain different visual elements. As he reflected, however, on the infinite wealth of colors of the rainbow, he could not believe that there could be a different visual element in the human retina for each of those many colors. He overcame this hurdle by a conclusion of sweeping import: the human retina must contain a very small number of visual elements—three, or possibly a few more. If there are three, he reasoned, each of the three will, when excited, produce the sensation of one of the three primary colors: red, or green, or blue. None of these visual elements is, however, restricted to perceiving one type of light; that particular type of light is merely the one to which it is most sensitive. If the eye is exposed to yellow light, all three visual elements are excited, each to a different degree, and the resultant blend of the three sensations is precisely what we call yellow (Fig. 28).

Young's theory was later expanded by Helmholtz into what we know as the Young-Helmholtz three-color theory, but for a long time it remained a hypothesis, impossible to prove by experimental evidence. Not until our own day did scientists furnish experimental proof. Chief among them was the Swedish scientist Granit. Unlike his precursors, Granit returned to animal experimentation and did all his work on the eye itself. This procedure guaranteed that the findings related to the eye, and not to the evaluating apparatus in the brain.

He used the electrophysiological method, recording the minute electric currents which are generated in a sensory nerve when a sense organ is stimulated. Figure

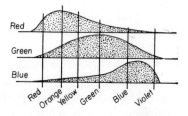

FIG. 28. Sensitivity of the three receptor systems of the human retina according to the Young-Helmholtz theory.

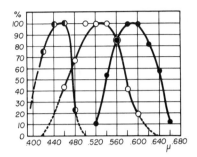

FIG. 29. Modulator curve of the cat. black, red; white, green; black-white, blue. Homoenergetic spectrum. (After Granit, 1945.)

29 shows what takes place. Just as the theory predicted, we see three separate curves, each of which relates to a specific type of cone; unlike the situation shown in Figure 28, these three curves overlap only slightly. This circumstance leads to certain difficulties which might be evaded by postulating the existence of a greater number of types of cone. Many modern scientists have assumed that there are four, five, or even as many as seven different types. Fundamentally, however, these modern experiments present an excellent confirmation of the old theory, for even Young did not insist rigidly on the number three. The three-color theory in its modern form is the foundation of our knowledge about color vision. Its most striking feature is the now-proven notion that each color, although homogeneous in itself and of a specific wave length, is divided by the eye into three parts; not until they reach the sensory center of the brain are the parts reassembled into a new entity.

This observation is reinforced by the remarkable fact that the eye cannot analyze a blend of colors into its components. The ear, on the other hand, can without difficulty distinguish the individual tones that compose a complex sound. The color sensation known as "greenish yellow" may be the product of (1) the pure greenish yellow of the spectrum, (2) a mixture of red and green, or (3) a mixture of orange and yellowish green. The physical composition of the light is different in each of these cases, and yet the human eye will see each as greenish yellow.

We now have some idea of the part the retina plays in our color vision. Next let us look at the function of the visual center of the human brain. The best approach to this problem should be through a study of what we call complementary colors. It has been known for some time that a great many pairs of colors will cancel each other out when they are seen together on a rapidly rotating color-disk. Bluish green and red, greenish yellow and violet, and many other such color pairs produce the impression of a neutral, colorless light. Humans are not the only creatures that perceive this remarkable phenomenon; something quite analogous has been demonstrated in fishes, bees, and water fleas.

This phenomenon, which seems to play so important a role in the color sense of every organism, is a mystery to the physicist. He is unable to explain why light of a wave length of 591 millimicrons and light of a wave length of 490 millimicrons are mutually antagonistic. It was believed for a while that chemistry would find the explanation. Certain substances are affected differently by light of a long wave length and light of a short wave length. The oxidation of sodium sulfate, for instance, is retarded by violet light, but accelerated by reddish yellow. If we assume that our visual cells contain substances endowed with properties similar to those of sodium sulfate, we have found a key to the mystery of complementary colors. This course was adopted by Ewald Hering in his famous theory, which ascribes "assimilatory" effects to one variety of light and "dissimilatory" effects to the other one—meaning that the two varieties of light are supposed to affect the metabolism of the light-sensitive cell in diametrically opposed fashions. This hypothesis, ingenious as it is, was abandoned long ago. Its flaw is that it attempts to explain the nature of the complementary colors through the activity of the visual cells. The accepted three-color theory affords no possibility for this.

Can any experiment demonstrate that the complementary colors do not originate in the retina, but in the brain? Those who study the laws of the mixing of colors usually watch the color-disk bearing the two complementary colors with both eyes simultaneously. This procedure, however, tells them nothing about where the mixing of the colors actually takes place—whether in the retina, in the nerve layer of the eye, or in the brain. There is, however, a simple experiment that is most revealing. Hold a piece of red glass in front of your left eye, and a piece of green glass in front of your right one, and look at a white surface (a piece of cloth will do). The result will be unexpected: the impressions will combine in your brain to produce a sensation of pure white which no longer shows any trace of the two components. The quest for the nature of the complementary colors thus comes to a remarkable end. The recognition that the intermingling of colors takes place in the depths of the brain, while constituting a great step forward in our knowledge, at the same time precludes the possibility of an exact physicochemical explanation. All that we have hoped to deduce from this experiment crumbles to nothing in our hands.

Black

Brown, ochre, vermilion, sap-green, ultramarine, and black lie side by side in peaceful harmony on the palette of the painter. No layman would think of making a distinction among these different colors. He might, at best, recognize a contrast between white or black and the other colors, by calling the other colors "bright" or "gay." All of them are "colors" to him. If you ask a physicist, he, however, will tell you that black does not belong in this gay company at all, not because it looks so somber, but because it is of an entirely different origin.

All the other colors on the palette send some type of light, or a mixture of various types of light, into the eyes of the onlooker. But "black" is the optical sensation caused by the absence of light. This is one of the strangest things in the world—just how strange becomes apparent if we try to think of an analogous experience in another sensory region. How would it strike you if in the midst of otherwise absolute silence you kept constantly hearing a certain sound that could never be heard under any other circumstances? Or if you kept smelling a peculiar odor whenever there was no smell? We could of course accustom ourselves to such a sensory world; it is by no means beyond the bounds of human imagination. But the most gifted storyteller could never make us envision a world in which there was no black. In such a world our faculty of vision would cease to exist at the boundary of a black area. What would we see, then, in that area itself? Nothing!

It is easy to realize that such a "nothing" cannot exist in our sensory world. The primary duty of our eyes is to give us an idea of the distribution in space of the objects around us. The space that surrounds us, despite its infinite extent, is a complete unit. There are no "holes," no gaps in it, for there is something wherever you may look. When there is no tree or bush or speck of soil to see, you see the vault of the sky, the clouds, or the stars winking at you from infinite distances. There is no room in this world for "nothing," and there can likewise be no visual sensation that would give us the illusion of seeing such "nothing." So we perceive the sensation known as "black" when no light impinges upon our eyes.

Another example will demonstrate that the human eye tolerates no gaps in its field of vision. There is a spot

FIG. 30. Experimental materials for demonstrating the blind spot. See text. (After Kühn.)

within the eye, the blind spot, situated where the optic nerve enters. Since the blind spot contains neither rods nor cones, we cannot see anything with it. Try this experiment: shut your left eye and hold Figure 30 before your right eye, staring fixedly at the white cross in the black field. Now take a kitchen match and hold it so that its head is directly in front of the cross. If you then shift the match toward the right, without taking your eye from the cross, the head of the match will disappear abruptly, to reappear as soon as your hand has moved a little farther to the right. At the spot where you saw nothing, the image of the head of the match fell right onto your blind spot. From this experiment the size, position, and shape of the blind spot can be calculated accurately (Fig. 31).

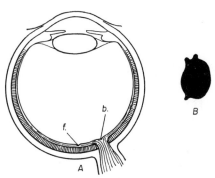

FIG. 31. *A*, a human eye. *f.*, the *fovea centralis*; *b.*, the blind spot. *B*, front view of the blind spot, more greatly magnified.

This simple physiological experiment demonstrates the existence of the blind spot. A person who never tried such an experiment and never read about it would live his life without ever becoming aware of this peculiar flaw. The reason for this ignorance is, of course, that we usually see with both eyes simultaneously. The constant co-operation of the eyes makes it impossible for a point to be projected onto both blind spots at the same time, so that we always see with at least one eye. Even when we use only one eye, there is still no perceptible evidence of the existence of the blind spot; where the blind spot should appear, the rods and cones situated around it take over. The rods and cones camouflage the blind spot with their own perceptions, thus preventing the formation of a hole in the field of vision.

This example demonstrates that our sense organs—at any rate our eyes—are far from being mechanical instruments. A mechanical instrument indicates with uncompromising accuracy whatever it is its duty to indicate. But the sense organs teach us a lesson of profound import—that truth is not of ultimate importance. Life is more important than truth, and this is why our sense organs are not uncompromising sticklers for truth, whenever the truth would result in harm to the organism. We shall discuss this point more specifically in the next chapter.

3. *The Adjustment of the Visual Images*

Because of the constant alternation of night and day, the light reflected by the objects in our environment varies widely. When the sun shines directly on a white-washed wall, the wall reflects many times more light than it does in the early morning or in the dull glow of dusk. If our eyes were mere mechanical instruments that reported with pedantic accuracy whatever was going on in the world about us, they would register the image of a dark gray wall in the morning, of a light gray wall a little later, and of a wall snow-white at high noon. In other words the same object would present itself, chameleon-like, in the widest variety of disguises. Such a chaotic situation would have a disastrous effect on our ability to recognize objects—practically the most important function of our eyes.

Adaptation

The constancy of visual images is mostly the result of what we call adaptation. In order to understand this process, it might help to recall the principles of the camera. When a photographer wants to take a picture, he must first check on the lighting conditions. If the illumination is too bright, he uses a narrower shutter opening and a shorter exposure time. If the light is dim, he compensates by using a longer exposure and opening the shutter as wide as possible. The eye produces the same effect by an adjustment of the pupil, which contracts when there is too much light and expands when the light is dim.

The adaptation of the pupil is overshadowed by the ability of the retina to adjust its sensitivity to great changes in the light. Think of a camera once again. When you want to photograph a dimly lit indoor scene, you use the most sensitive film available, but you use a less sensitive one for taking outdoor pictures in strong sunlight. Nature follows the same procedure; to distinguish this process from the mechanical adaptation of the pupil of the eye, we call it physiological adaptation.

Physiological adaptation is by no means an exclusive property of the complicated human optical apparatus. The same process operates in animals that have only a cutaneous light sense and can do no more than distinguish "brighter" from "dimmer."

How can such subtle facts be proven? Let us experiment with a barnacle. As soon as the light dims, this creature retreats into its solid shell. If we put the barnacle in artificial light which we can measure in units, we can determine what reduction in the light will provoke this reaction. The most convenient unit of measurement is the lux, which equals one meter-candle. The answer may be 5 lux; in other words, if we reduce the illumination from 100 to 95 lux, the timid little creature will retreat into its shell instantly, while in a light of 96 lux the barnacle will stay outside. Our next step is to condition the barnacle to the dim light of only 10 lux. We shall then observe a distinct reaction when we dim that light by as little as half a lux, from 10 to 9.5. Whereas in the previous experiment the animal displayed no reaction at all to a reduction of 4 lux, it now reacts immediately to a reduction of .5 lux. Its exposure to the feeble illumination has made it ten times as sensitive.

White and gray

Adaptation is not the only device for keeping visual images constant under different conditions. Since a dimly illuminated white and a brightly illuminated gray reflect the same amount of white light, a physicist makes no distinction between them. To our eyes, however, white and gray will never look like the same color.

The experiment to demonstrate this is a very simple one. Take a piece of gray paper in your hand, and stand with your back to the window, so that the paper catches the daylight from outside. Now look past the paper at a dimly lit white wall. If you rely on some physical apparatus—say, a photographic camera—to decide which object is lighter, the answer will be that the paper is much lighter, for it reflects many times the amount of light reflected by the wall. But if you consult your eyes the verdict will be totally different: they will assure you that the paper is gray but brightly lit, whereas the wall is white but dimly lit.

This experience demonstrates that the human eye is incomparably superior to any mechanical apparatus, regardless of how intricate the latter may be. The apparatus records things, the eye interprets them. But it is very easy to reduce the human eye to the level of a machine. All you have to do is punch a small hole in a piece of cardboard and look through it at the two objects in turn. When your eye cannot compare the object and its surroundings, you will conclude that the wall is darker than the piece of gray paper.

Flatfish have eyes which to some extent interpret rather than simply record data. These fish blend in completely with their background; when they lie on sand, they look quite light, and when on darker ground, darker. Yet when they swim about, they manage to maintain the same color under the most diverse lighting conditions. How do they do it? The skin of their backs contains pigment cells which are controlled by a reflex starting in the eyes. Researchers have ascertained that such a fish perceives the ratio between the light shining from above and that reflected from below. Since this ratio remains constant for one spot during the entire day, the color of the fish, which is geared to this ratio, remains the same while the fish swims about.

The adjustment of size

Our eyes trick us, to our advantage, not only as regards the brightness of visual images, but also as to their sizes. If the eye were simply a mechanical apparatus, the farther it was from an object the smaller it would show that object to be; but the brain, which translates the retinal images into sensations, corrects their apparent sizes.

Your two hands are all the experimental equipment you need to study this phenomenon. If you look at one of your hands first at close range and then at arm's length, you will experience a remarkable illusion. Your hand will appear to be the same size in both instances, even though its retinal image is bound to be substantially smaller in the second instance. You can readily understand how this miracle comes to pass if you compare your hands while holding one of them close to your eyes and the other at a distance, shifting your gaze back and forth from one hand to the other. As long as you keep both eyes open, your hands look exactly the same size, but if you close one eye you will suddenly find yourself gazing at two hands of very different sizes. The illusion of equal size was obviously due to the fact that you looked with both eyes at the same time. When both eyes are trained on an object, the angle at which the two visual axes come together is communicated to the brain by the many sensory endings in the eye muscles. The nearer the observed object is to the eyes, the more obtuse is the angle of convergence. From the angle of convergence the brain is able to determine how many times the retinal image must be enlarged.

The adjustment of visual images is not restricted to close-range vision. To test this statement, take a look at the wallpaper in your room. You will realize that no matter how much the light changes, or how far you are from the wall, you still see the same pattern. The design of the wallpaper—suppose it is three red roses surrounded by green leaves—appears the same size whether you look at it from a distance of three feet or six feet. Now focus both your eyes sharply on your right thumb and hold the thumb so that you see the roses right next to it. Since your eyes are adjusted to close-range vision, the roses will shrivel to quite a tiny image. Here, as in the experiment with your hands, your gauging of distance is responsible for the apparent sizes of the objects. When the eyes are focused on objects at varying distance, the angle of convergence permits the brain to adjust the size. When the eyes are focused only on the near object—the thumb —the brain does not pay sufficient attention to the pattern on the wallpaper to adjust its size, and it therefore appears tiny.

The phenomenon of adjustment naturally ceases when

the distance is great. As we look along a tree-lined avenue which extends all the way to the horizon, even if the trees are all the same height the more distant ones look smaller to us. Although the adjustment of visual images presents illusions at close and middle ranges, one is subject to considerable illusions in looking at things at long distances. Adults have usually learned to disregard these illusions, but a child must amass a great deal of experience before he can understand that a man he sees crossing the street one hundred yards away is not a tiny dwarf from fairyland, but a grownup of normal size.

4. The Sense of Hearing

When you feel an urge to get away from the burden of daily living, from the constant rush and noise of city life, the best escape is to return for a while to nature. Whether you retreat to the solitude of the lofty mountains, to the cool, green forests, or visit the sunlit fields and meadows, you will find everywhere in nature a tonic: the stillness which permits you to listen to the sound of your own breathing. If you are seated at the edge of a forest on a calm, windless summer evening, only now and then will the call of a pheasant, a noise made by a frightened roebuck, the raucous screech of a bird of prey, or the chirping of the crickets in the meadow break the silence.

Of all the noises heard in nature, those which have the strongest effect on human emotions are spoken in the powerful language of the elements: the howling of the wind, the roar of a waterfall, the roll of thunder. Animals, which are more practical creatures, evaluate sounds differently. They are indifferent to elemental sounds and attend only noises produced by another animal—a call, a cry, a screech, or animal movements. In animals, therefore, the ability to utter sounds and the sense of hearing are usually interlinked; one exists for the sake of the other.

Song and love

The preceding statement should not, of course, be taken to mean that all animals have one common language by which they can communicate with one another, as they do in fairy tales. It simply means that every animal is attracted chiefly by the sounds emitted by another member of its own kind. Originally, before it became a tool of communication among members of a species, the voice was used solely to attract the female to the male. The language of love was thus the first language in the world, and the first ear in the world was created for the sole purpose of hearing the amorous chirping or screeching of some romantic suitor. From such limited use, the ear and the voice of man and the higher animals became ever more versatile tools of communication—so much so that, Caruso notwithstanding, we no longer have any inkling of their original significance, and we must learn it anew from the crickets and the frogs.

The frogs, the crickets, the grasshoppers, and the cicadas present the problem in its simplest form. Among these creatures only the males usually have the gift of song. This fact was known to Aristophanes, that unchivalrous Greek poet of antiquity, who wrote, "Happy lives the crickets lead, for they have mute wives." The females are mute but interested listeners. When they hear the song of a male, the females obey an irresistible compulsion to leave their haunts and hurry to him, so that one singer is sometimes surrounded by a whole bevy of female admirers. We know that the sense of hearing and vocal development are both linked closely to love life in these creatures because the males vie with one another in this remarkable singing competition only in the courting season. Yet it seems to have direct relationship to the act of courting. Is it an expression of joy or a challenge to competition? Its exact purpose is as yet unknown.

An increasing severance of the links between voice and hearing on the one hand and love life on the other is observable among the higher vertebrates. At the other end of the scale, our study cannot begin below the evolutionary level of the birds, because most reptiles (snakes, lizards, turtles) are deaf and dumb. Snakes are totally deaf. The musical instruments used by the snake charmers in India are mere stage props, designed to deceive the audience. Nor can any noise or sound in this world ever disturb the serene calm of the turtles. Though untold effort and patience was expended in experiments attempting to persuade these creatures that they can hear something if they only want to. A well-developed sense of hearing is possessed only by the crocodiles, which are also able to bellow in the rutting season.

Among the birds the mating song of the male is, naturally, the most important use of the voice; in many species the females do not sing. Many gullible bird fanciers learn this fact to their grief when the canary bought as a male turns out later to be a nonsinging female.

Let us now consider the mammals, the highest group on the scale of evolution. To be sure, even mammals occasionally show some evidence of a close link between the use of the voice and sex life—an example is the mating call of the deer. Even this case, however, shows a substantial shift of purpose since the primary objective of the buck's vocal display is to hurl a challenge at his rival. Nor can the awful caterwauling of lovesick cats be construed as a love song designed to attract the female, for both mates join voices in the concert. Except for these cases of vocal display, which are for purposes other than attracting the female, the link between voice and love life has been completely eliminated. A great many mammals are practically mute; only the fear of death will make a rabbit emit its pitiful cry. Gregarious mammals, such as the marmot and the prairie dog, use their voices to warn their fellows when some danger is approaching. Still others, such as the lion, use their powerful voices to panic and scatter a herd of intended victims. The voice of many mammals is the expression of an inner excitement which also serves, like the spine-chilling roar of the big beasts of prey, to terrify the opponent.

If we survey all animals endowed with the ability to hear, we conclude that the evolution of the sense of hearing contrasts with that of the sense of sight. When we studied the sense of sight, we found that the lowest organisms reacted only to sunlight; in higher organisms the sun began to share its role as a stimulus with light reflected from objects, but only the highest organisms could perceive shapes sufficiently well to enable them to identify other organisms. On the other hand, only the lowest organisms use the sense of hearing exclusively for communication with other organisms, whereas in man the sense of hearing is stimulated by all sorts of other sounds.

The organs of hearing

Since the original purpose of the sense of hearing was to enable an organism to hear the love songs of a wooer, we would expect this sense to develop only when the organism could produce its own sounds. With a few exceptions, this is true of only two groups of animals: the insects and the terrestrial mammals. Let us therefore first discuss the organs of hearing in these two groups.

In both insects and terrestrial mammals, the method of breathing is related to the processes we are studying: in mammals, the faculty linked with breathing is that of the production of sounds, whereas in insects it is the ability to hear sounds. The voices of frogs, birds, and human beings are produced by squeezing air out of the lungs; in the larynx, this air sweeps past the vocal cords and makes them vibrate. Even animals which are otherwise totally mute may produce sounds in this fashion. A whale stranded on solid land will slowly choke to death because the weight of its body makes it impossible for it to breathe. As it tries to ventilate its lungs it will emit a moan audible for a great distance.

Certain insects produce their "song" by rubbing their hard wings together; others rub a hind leg, equipped with a special stridulatory organ, against a wing. But their ability to hear is linked essentially with the fact that they breathe through a system of air pipes called tracheae, which run through every part of their body. The tracheae widen at many places to form spacious air pockets, and these air pockets make possible the formation of a tympanic membrane (Fig. 32). Such a tympanic membrane is found wherever a true sense of hearing has evolved. Essentially, it is like the diaphragm of a telephone transmitter, and its function is similar: to vibrate in response to sounds.

In the simplest form of the organ of hearing, the auditory cells may lie directly on the tympanic membrane and be solidly attached to it (Fig. 32). In such a case, the cells vibrate along with the tympanic membrane. The "ear" of the grasshopper is of this variety, and so are also the auditory organs of cicadas and butter-

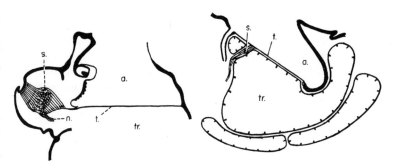

FIG. 32. Cross-section of the auditory organ of a cicada (left) and of a grasshopper (right). *s.*, sensory cells; *t.*, tympanic membrane; *tr.*, tracheal vesicle; *a.*, external air; *n.*, nerve.

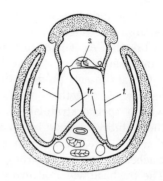

FIG. 33. Cross-sectional view of the foreleg of a locust with auditory organ. *s.*, sensory cell; *t.*, tympanic membrane; *tr.*, tracheal vesicles.

flies. The conduction of sound is more complicated in locusts and in vertebrates; in these animals the tympanic membrane vibrates independently, without reference to the sensory cells. Much deeper in the inner ear is a second membrane which receives the vibrations of the first one. This second membrane is the one to which the auditory cells are attached.

This complication is obviously a structural improvement. The outer tympanic membrane, especially when it is on the outer skin as in frogs or grasshoppers, can be excited by some mechanical stimulus, such as pressure or impact, when there is no sound. If the auditory cells are attached to it directly, an auditory reaction must ensue. But if the sensory cells are in contact only with the inner membrane, all mechanical impacts are limited to the tympanic membrane, and only genuine sound vibrations are conveyed to the inner membrane. It is easy to locate the site of this true acoustic membrane in the locusts. A cross-sectional view of the auditory organ of a locust—situated, strange as it may seem, in the forelegs of the insect—shows that the auditory cells are on the wall of one of the large air-conducting tracheae running lengthwise through the leg (Fig. 33).

Human beings present a more complicated picture. The auditory organs of humans and other mammals lie imbedded deep in the bony mass of the skull, so well concealed that it took scientists a long time to find them. The cochlea, the remarkable bony structure which houses the organ, was identified in 1561, but almost three full centuries passed before the great research scientist Alfonso Corti discovered the real sense organ, which later was named "organ of Corti" in his honor (Fig. 34). A cross-section of the cochlea shows three large spaces separated from each other by two membranes, with a third membrane located in the middle space. Reissner's membrane, which extends from one wall to the other, is of microscopic thinness; the basilar membrane carries the organ of Corti, a highly intricate structure of cells forming a vault, with the sensory cells inserted into that vault. Finally, above the sensory cells and in closest contact with the delicate sensory hairs, lies the so-called tectorial membrane (*membrana tectoria*).

We are free to choose which of these three membranes to credit with the ability to conduct sounds. Until very recently, the basilar membrane was the general

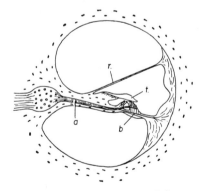

FIG. 34. Cross-section of the human cochlea. *b.*, basilar membrane; *r.*, Reissner's membrane; *t.*, tectorial membrane; *a.*, auditory nerve. (From Bütschli.)

choice for two obvious reasons: its close spatial relationship to the sensory cells, and its physical structure, which resembles a piano. If you stretch this membrane you find that it is really not a homogeneous membrane at all, but is composed of 24,000 taut fibers which run in parallels diagonally across the cochlea. The most interesting detail, however, is that these fibers are not of equal length; their length increases progressively from the base of the cochlea toward its apex, the longest ones being about eight times as long as the shortest.

As everybody who has studied physics knows, the specific rate of vibration of a rod depends on its length. Nothing could therefore be more logical than to assume that each such group of fibers of a certain length is intended to vibrate in unison with the particular note to which those fibers are attuned.

The resonance theory

The assumption above is the basis of the famous resonance theory of Helmholtz, which was until recently regarded as the best founded of all the hypotheses. No other theory can explain as smoothly and as elegantly the ability of the human ear to analyze sounds. As we know, the science of acoustics distinguishes tones, sounds,

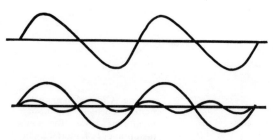

FIG. 35. Analysis of a sound composed of a fundamental tone and upper partials. (After Bunge.)

and noises. Physically, a tone is a manifestation of a sound wave of a definite frequency; the graphic representation of this frequency is a regular curve, called a sine curve. Although the graphic representation of what we call a sound likewise shows a completely periodic structure, the individual vibration deviates from the shape of the sine curve to a major or minor degree. It has been proved mathematically and confirmed by physical experimentation that every sound can be analyzed and dissected into a series of individual tones (Fig. 35). In this analysis the physicist uses resonators (hollow bodies which respond solely to their own specific tones). He notices which resonators begin to vibrate when a particular tone is sounded. But even without the aid of physics many people can hear the individual component tones of a complex sound and can distinguish the fundamental tones, upper partials, and so forth.

Although this seems to bear out the resonance theory of Helmholtz, several facts argue against it. To cite an example supplied by comparative physiology: even though the hearing of a parrot is in all likelihood as good as that of a human being, a parrot's basilar membrane contains only 1,200 fibers, whereas the corresponding membrane of a human ear contains 24,000. Fish have no basilar membranes at all, and yet they are capable of analyzing sounds.

Even more significant than these arguments, however, are certain recent experiments performed on the human ear. These experiments support the theory that, although a specific tone produces vibrations only in one spot of the membrane, this condition is not due to any specific attunement of the individual fibers, but to the presence of stationary waves in the inner ear. Two important points may be noted concerning these waves. Reissner's membrane, rather than the basilar membrane, plays an important part in their generation; and their dependence frequency is demonstrated by the fact that the higher

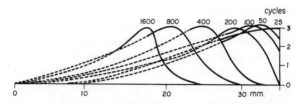

FIG. 36. The site of the amplitude of the vibration of the cochlear wall for sine-shaped vibrations of different frequencies. (After von Bekesy.)

the frequency, the nearer to the oval window does the stationary wave reach its maximum. This is clearly demonstrated in Figure 36.

The sense of hearing of bats

Scientists have recently taken particular interest in the sense of hearing of bats, moths, and fish. The sense of hearing of the bats is not a new subject. The Italian scholar Lazzaro Spallanzani noted in the late eighteenth century that blinded bats could skillfully avoid wires and other obstacles while flying about. His friend Jurine, of Geneva, found that the accuracy of the flight of the bats was seriously impaired if their ears were plugged; this circumstance led him to conclude, quite correctly, that bats became aware of obstacles through their sense of hearing. But only in the past decades was this problem taken up anew and solved at last.

Bats are skilled aerial navigators; they do their navigating according to the same principle which the human inventor of the sonic depth finder discovered scarcely more than thirty years ago. While a bat is airborne—and when it is preparing for a take-off—its larynx sends out rapid, rhythmic bursts of ultrasonics of a frequency so very high (from 40,000 to 80,000 vibrations a second) as to be completely inaudible to human ears. The wave length of ultrasonics is just a few millimeters, so that they are reflected even by small objects. The bat, catching these reflected sound waves with its big ears, is capable of truly amazing feats. It can determine the exact location of a tiny bug held before it in a pair of tweezers, it can find every crack that will offer it a foothold in a wall, and it can distinguish a piece of velvet from a piece of paper. In short, a bat can accomplish with its ears almost the same things that we can with our eyes.

The sense of hearing of moths

The sense of hearing of moths parallels that of the bats in an amazing fashion. This highly developed sense has long puzzled naturalists, for since practically all these insects are voiceless their sense of hearing could not possibly be an auxiliary of their sex life. Another intriguing point is the fact that while auditory organs are found in certain types of moths, such organs are completely missing from the moths' diurnal cousins, the butterflies.

Today we know that by endowing certain moths with a sense of hearing, Nature gave them a potent defense against their most dangerous enemies, the bats. The tiny auditory organs of the moths are attuned to the pitch of the ultrasonics emitted by the bats, and they may react to those short waves in several characteristic ways. If a moth is airborne when he detects a bat's ultrasonics, he will either about-face in mid-air, like a frightened rabbit, or will plummet straight down to the ground to find a hiding place; if he hears the ultrasonics just as he is preparing for a take-off, he will simply delay his flight and stay quietly where he is.

The sense of hearing of fish

The ancients studied this question. In fact, it was reported by Pliny that Marcus Crassus, the fat man who was the partner of Pompey and Julius Caesar in the

triumvirate that ruled the Roman Empire, had a tame
eel which on hearing his call would obediently swim up
to him and eat out of his hand. Similar reports—which,
naturally, are devoid of all value as scientific proof—
have appeared in modern times. A famous incident is the
exposure of the secret of the "hearing fish" of the
Kremsmünster monastery. These fish were reputed to
swim to their feeding place whenever a bell was sounded,
but a Viennese naturalist demonstrated that if the fish
could not see the man who pulled the bell cord they
paid no attention to the sound of the bell.

After the fame of the Kremsmünster fish had faded, it
was shown by Emil Du Bois-Reymond that many fish
will not react at all to sounds powerful enough to hurt
human ears. He constructed a special musical instrument in which an electromagnet caused a steel plate,
about 17 inches in width, to make a horrible racket. He
submerged this apparatus in the water, turned it on, and
observed the behavior of the fish in its vicinity. Observing the fish was, of course, no simple job. The observer had to get in the pool and swim around the plate.
He noted two things: first that he, himself, was hardly
able to bear the racket, and second that the fish paid no
attention to it at all.

All the evidence tends to bear out the contention that
fish in their normal habitat pay absolutely no attention
to sound. After what we have learned about the biological
significance of the sense of hearing in other primitive
forms of animal life, it seemed unlikely that they would.
The majority of fish are totally mute, and since they are
unable to communicate with other members of their
species "by word of mouth," why should they pay any
attention to sounds? Despite this logic and the experiments which seemed to disprove the existence of a
sense of hearing in fish, science eventually adopted a
different point of view. Today we know that fish do
have a sense of hearing—in fact, a fairly acute one.

The mystery was solved, as in many other cases, by an experiment involving careful training and conditioning. One could argue that the fat triumvir Crassus, and the monks of Kremsmünster, must have trained their fish too, but there is all the difference in the world between those early cases and modern experimental techniques. Another argument might be that Du Bois-Reymond proved beyond all doubt that fish will not react to sound. Again, there is a vast difference between a stimulus applied in a random fashion, which means nothing to the animal, and a meaningful one. A stimulus becomes meaningful when the animal associates it with another fact. Experiments with meaningful stimuli gave astonishing results: if a fish receives its food only when a certain note is sounded, the otherwise uninteresting sound becomes significant to the fish. Systematic conditioning experiments show that fish can hear under water just as well as a human being, that they have what we call "absolute pitch," and that they can distinguish slight intervals and hear a specific note within a complex tone (tone analysis). As a matter of fact, there is only one

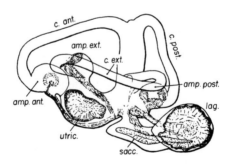

FIG. 37. Right labyrinth of a minnow, seen from within. *amp. ant., amp. ext.* and *amp. post.*, the three ampullae. *c. ant., c. ext.* and *c. post.* are the three semicircular canals. *utric.*, utriculus. *sacc.*, sacculus. *lag.*, lagena. (After von Frisch.)

point in which the human sense of hearing is superior to that of the fish: the localization of sounds. This faculty is very poorly developed in fish.

The study of the organ of hearing in fish has led to remarkable findings. Fish have no organ equivalent to the organ of Corti, located in the human cochlea. Instead the saccule, that part of the labyrinth where in a human ear the cochlea begins, has evolved into the organ of hearing (Fig. 37). In many species of fish, that part of the labyrinth which serves the sense of equilibrium and that part which functions as the auditory organ (the utricle and the saccule) are so distant from each other that they can be removed by separate surgical operations. A fish deprived of its utricle seems to "stagger" as it swims, but it can still be conditioned to respond to sounds. On the other hand, a fish without its saccule retains its normal equilibrium in swimming, but is no longer able to hear. This means that the saccule and the adjacent lagena constitute the auditory organ of the fish.

Many varieties of fishes, belonging to many different families, have been found to possess a good sense of hearing. One group is especially notable: the Ostariophysi, which include the cyprinoid fish (members of the carp family) as well as the sheatfish. The Ostariophysi, strangely enough, use their air bladders as instruments of hearing (Fig. 38). The saccule links the air bladder with the organ of Weber, which consists of three small bones, arranged in a single line behind each other; the largest one, the malleus, is the rearmost of the three and touches the air bladder, while the smallest one, the stapes, occupies the foremost position and ends at a canal-like bulge of the saccule. Sound waves pervade the entire body of the fish and cause a vibration of the air in the air bladder. These vibratory impulses are transmitted by the ossicles of Weber to the liquid of the saccule. The removal of the air bladder of such a fish causes a substantial impairment of its hearing.

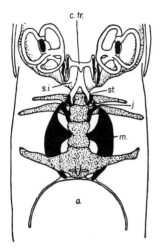

FIG. 38. Ostariophysi. The drawing shows the linkage of the air bladder and the labyrinth through the ossicles of Weber (in black). *m.*, malleus; *j.*, incus; *st.*, stapes; *s.i.*, sinus impair; *c. tr.*, *canalis transversus*; *a.*, air bladder. (After von Frisch.)

5. *Smell and Taste*

Many varieties of animal life have no sense of hearing; many, especially among the lower orders, have no perception of light. But nowhere in this world is there a form of animal life that does not react to some chemical stimuli. The universality of the chemical sense is perhaps explained by the fact that in order to eat the organism must possess some chemical knowledge. After all, even the lowly amoeba, crawling sluggishly on the bottom of a stagnant pool, must be able to distinguish a grain of sand from an alga or some other digestible form of life, or else it would starve to death.

The purposes of the chemical sense, however, go far beyond the mere selection of food. Life in this world manifests itself in an almost infinite number of forms and varieties. Each of the innumerable species of animal, plant, or bacterium has its own specific smell. Just recall the unique scent emitted by the blossoms, leaves, and fruits of various plants. Bacteria have no specific odor of their own, but they usually create an intense smell through their metabolic products, as we have discovered by personal experience with cheese, rotting carcasses, and so on. Even the smell of one's native soil comes from the bacteria that live in it. And finally, among the higher animals, odor is not limited to skunks and goats. Even animals that have no specific odor perceptible to humans almost always identify themselves by their smell to members of their own species or to other animals with which they have a biological relation. We find therefore that in addition to gustation (the perception of taste stimuli), another fundamental function of the chemical sense is olfaction (the perception and recognition of smells).

In two highly developed forms of animal life, the vertebrates and the insects, the sense of taste and the sense of smell can be completely divorced from each other and regarded as two distinct, mutually independent senses. Man smells with his nose and tastes with his tongue. In all vertebrates the olfactory nerve runs in the most frontal position from the nose to the central nervous system, while the fifth, seventh, and ninth cranial nerves conduct the gustatory stimulation of the tongue to the brain (Fig. 39). This clear evidence of the separation of these senses is corroborated by physiological experiment. If we remove the entire forebrain of a fish it can no longer smell, but it can still be conditioned to respond to taste stimuli.

The study of the insects reveals a similar separation. A bee perceives smells with its long antennae, but tastes with its mouth parts. As a result, these two spatially separate senses can be severed from each other by amputation of the bee's antennae. No one has ever succeeded in performing such an experiment on other forms of animal life—worms, snails, mollusks, and so forth. A crayfish, for instance, perceives smells with its antennae, but if the antennae are amputated, it can still smell. The

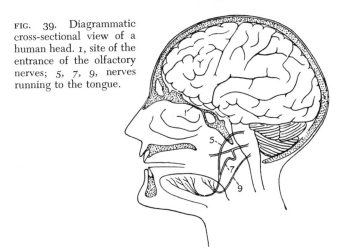

FIG. 39. Diagrammatic cross-sectional view of a human head. *1*, site of the entrance of the olfactory nerves; *5, 7, 9,* nerves running to the tongue.

explanation is that in addition to these appendages, the crayfish has olfactory cells in its mouth parts, and perhaps in the gill chamber.

From these findings scientists have leapt to the conclusion that animals of this sort have but one indivisible chemical sense. Is this view warranted? Not in my opinion! It is true that in these animals the sensory cells of smell and taste are situated so closely together that they cannot be successfully separated by operation. But the evidence from anatomy and physiology does not allow us to assume that the senses are identical because the organs are not separated. In the following discussion we shall therefore take it for granted that these two chemical senses exist separately in every member of the animal kingdom. First let us consider the sense of smell.

Olfaction and sex life

How the mating partners of the various animal species find each other is one of the most fascinating and important questions of biology. All life on earth would have become extinct a long time ago but for the factors which enable every animal to find a sexual partner during its mating season. As we know, the male animals are supposed to seek out the females; in many species, this is their only purpose in life. For gregarious animals (here we include humans), finding a mate is not a difficult feat, but the great majority of both land and water animals lead completely solitary lives; for these animals the mating season is the only time when the paths of two members of the same species cross. Take a moth for example. The caterpillar spends its entire life in solitude on the plant which supplies it with food, indifferent to anything but eating its fill; during the period of pupation, when it burrows under the surface of the soil, it is even more isolated than before. But when the male moth bursts from his cocoon in the spring, he must immediately seek out a female of his own species and mate with her. How does he accomplish this?

If you take a walk in the woods on a summer night, countless moths will soon be buzzing about you. There are hundreds of different moths, all of which look alike to a layman, and often even an expert finds it difficult to tell them apart. Their incredibly fine sense of smell is the only thing that enables them to know the members of their own species with absolute certainty in all that multitude. Each female moth emits a very delicate scent which is unique to her species. This scent is so subtle, so delicate, that a human being is unable to perceive it

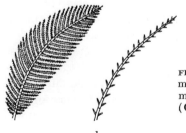

FIG. 40. Antennae of *a*, a male and *b*, a female moth, *Saturnia pavonia*. (Original.)

a   *b*

even if the tiny creature is held right next to his nose. When one considers that the atmosphere of the entire forest must be saturated with hundreds of such odors, the difficulty of the task of the male becomes apparent. But despite these seemingly insurmountable difficulties, the male moth with his enormous antennae (Fig. 40) is amazingly quick in finding a mate.

Collectors take advantage of this ability of the male moth, which offers them the surest and easiest way to catch the males of many species, especially the silkworms. All you need for this purpose is a female that has just emerged from the cocoon. Put her in a small gauze cage and take her at night to a place frequented by males of her species. Although you may have to wait for a while until the first swain arrives, he will soon be followed by a host of others. Males can even be attracted through an open window in a big city. A female of some common species will often attract dozens of male moths into the room.

Although scientists have no positive proof as yet, there can be little doubt that most of the other lower animals, such as snails and earthworms, also find their mating partners by relying solely on the sense of smell. How else could they do it? They cannot see, and it is practically inconceivable that two closely related snails, distinguishable only by a difference in the designs of their shells, could tell by their sense of touch whether the other is of the same species or just a distant cousin.

Sea urchins do not mate at all. The entire "sex life" of the male and female sea urchin consists of ejecting the sperm and the eggs into the sea water at the same time. The spermatozoids then swim about and fertilize whatever eggs they happen to meet. But even this process, simple as it is, must be controlled and directed by the chemical sense. It would be useless for a male sea urchin to release his sperm when there were no eggs in the vicinity, for the spermatozoids would soon be carried away and scattered by the waves. In order to prevent such an occurrence, a certain substance (about which we know very little) is released into the water along with the sex cells. This substance acts as a signal to every sea urchin of the opposite sex that the time has come to follow suit. Thus, when one sea urchin starts the process, there is a chain reaction: whole clouds of whitish sperm and transparent ova are simultaneously ejected into the water in the same vicinity, giving the two elements a very good chance of being united.

Things are quite different among the higher forms of animal life. For the birds, the sense of smell has no sexual-biological importance; their song is the principal instrument that brings the two sexes together, and they recognize one another by their feathers. Among the highest animals, the mammals, smell once again becomes a factor of paramount importance. It takes no profound learning to see this. It is a fact of everyday life that a male dog recognizes a female dog by her smell. Clever burglars are said to take advantage of this fact: before attempting to invade a home guarded by a fierce male dog, they rub on themselves the scent of a female dog, so that the watchdog does not receive them with menacing fangs, but with its tail wagging a friendly welcome.

Friend and foe

In addition to leading the male animal to the female of its species, the chemical sense also enables most animals to tell friend from foe. Lower animals make this distinction without any conscious reference to previous experience, by virtue of their ancient heritage of instincts. For such a purpose, the superiority of the chemical sense to the other senses is quite obvious. When an enemy intends to make a meal out of you, you cannot expect to examine him by leisurely feeling his body with your tactile organs. The sense of touch is obviously unsuited for this purpose, and the sense of sight is far too poorly developed in most animals of the lower orders to do them any good in this kind of situation. This leaves only the chemical sense, which does the job well. The mussels and snails instinctively flee as soon as they smell a starfish, their natural enemy. We have already observed the way a scallop notices anything that moves (p. 62). Fish make very shrewd and versatile use of the sense of smell to deal appropriately with friend and foe. Among the gregarious fish, such as the minnows, the "tribal scent" probably helps to keep the school together. The sense of smell of the minnows gives them, in addition, twofold protection against their natural enemies, the predatory fish. If a minnow is seized by a pike, the minnow's injured skin discharges a substance which warns the rest of the school of the danger. As soon as the other minnows receive the warning signal they take to flight. But minnows can also identify the pike itself by its scent. When the small defenseless fish catch this scent, they rarely attempt flight, for this would bring no escape from the fast marauder. Instead they usually become totally motionless and sink slowly to the bottom. This is an extraordinarily practical expedient, because the pike is "sight-guided" and reacts chiefly to anything that moves.

The detection of food

Finding food is no problem for us; we just go to a store and buy some. Yet occasionally we revert to our natural state and actually search for food on our own. Every one of us must have passed pleasant hours picking strawberries, blueberries, or mushrooms in thickets. We have no need of our noses for picking berries, since their red and blue hues beckon us invitingly.

The mushrooms, however, are not always so obliging. The delicious truffles hide underground, in the shadow of spreading oaks, and the nose is the only sense organ that can find them. Since man's own nose is not keen enough for the job, he has to depend upon the nose of an animal—usually a pig. The truffle hunter puts a collar around the neck of a pig and leads the animal to a meadow where big oaks grow; then he waits expectantly while the pig, led by its acute sense of smell, digs in the ground. As soon as the pig has pulled up a truffle and is ready to devour it, the man shoves a club between the pig's jaws and puts the truffle into his own pocket.

Man and pig are thus representative of the two principal types of food-hunters: the sight-guided and the scent-guided animals. Among the mammals—the pig, the dog, the bear, the hedgehog, the shrew, to name just a few of the many thousands of species—the scent-guided type predominates. Primates and cats are the only sight-guided mammals, but the whole class of birds is sight-guided. Both types also occur among the lower vertebrates. Frogs and pikes, for instance, are sight-guided, whereas salamanders and eels are scent-guided. Among the invertebrates, the degree to which the eyes are developed is in inverse proportion to the sense of smell. On the evolutionary level of the insects, the purely sight-guided type is rare; the dragonfly is its only notable representative. As for crayfish, snails, and worms, we can say that their eyes play no part whatsoever in their search for food.

The bats constitute a unique group; as we have seen, they track down their prey with the aid of their sense of hearing.

The sharpness of the sense of smell

In studying the sense of smell, we humans are handicapped by the poor quality of our own. Very few animals can excel our senses of sight and hearing but we must confess we are miserable dullards when it comes to olfaction. We and our cousins, the monkeys and apes, constitute the group of "microsmatics" (creatures with a poor sense of smell), whereas dogs, bears, deer, and a great many other animals are "macrosmatics"

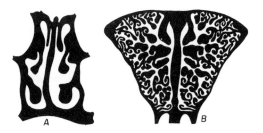

FIG. 41. Sketch of the cross-sectional views of the rear part of the nasal cavity of two mammals. *A*, a microsmatic mammal (man); *B*, a macrosmatic mammal (deer). (After von Frisch.)

(endowed with a keen sense of smell). The cross-sectional views of the two different types of noses is eloquent evidence of this sad truth (Fig. 41).

Even though we stand on the bottom rung of the ladder of olfactory ability, the sensitivity of the human nose nevertheless borders on the incredible. Chemical reagents used for detecting substances which emit odor are not nearly as accurate as the mucous membrane of the human nose. For example, the nose of a human being is able to detect the smell of 1/1,000,000 of one milligram of vanillin in one liter of air. If you express these microscopic quantities as numbers of molecules, however, you will find that even those figures are of astronomical proportions. The smallest number of molecules of formic acid detectable in 50 cc. of air is 1.6×10^{16} (that is, 16 quadrillion); of chloroform, 7.6×10^{15} (that is, 7.6 quintillion).

Although we are aware of the acuity of a dog's sense of smell, just *what* a dog smells is bound to remain unknown to us. The ability of a dog to pick out the specific scent of a certain person from among many other similar scents seems remarkable to us. The dog will not only identify the track of its master, but the crisscrossing tracks of different dogs. Another amazing fact is that a well-trained dog can pick out from among several similar pieces of wood the one that a certain person has held in his hand—even if the person had washed his hands before handling the wood, and had held the wood for only two seconds.

Similar feats can be expected from the other macrosmatic mammals. But insects are capable of even more incredible discriminations. I shall not go into the details of how male butterflies seek out their females over great distances, but shall briefly mention an insect less known to us—the Ephialtes wasp.

Since the eggs of the Ephialtes wasp can thrive only when embedded in the body of a living creature, the mother wasp searches for a live animal in which to deposit her eggs. Most of the time she chooses the larva of some other insect. Flitting from one cabbage to another all day long, the mother wasp is bound to find a victim exposed on a leaf—for example, a caterpillar of the cabbage butterfly. Some of the exploring Ephialtes wasps, however, look specifically for larvae of creatures that spend their lives concealed deep in wood—creatures such as the wood wasp, which can gnaw through the thickest boards. A man would have a hard time finding such a larva, as it lies deep under the bark of pines and

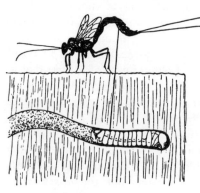

FIG. 42. An Ephialtes wasp injecting its egg into a wood-wasp larva hidden in a piece of wood. (After Doflein.)

firs. The Ephialtes wasp, however, uses the long antennae that are its organs of smell to explore a likely-looking tree. For a long time it scurries back and forth, constantly moving its antennae. When it finally finds the right spot, it raises its abdomen in a steep arch and places its ovipositor, a needle-sharp drill, against the bark. By carefully moving back and forth, it quickly drills a hole through the bark and the wood and into the soft body of the larva, which remains ignorant of its peril even as the death-dealing egg slides down into its body (Fig. 42)

Other Ephialtes wasps wage war against the mischief-making beetle *Tenebrio molitor,* which lies so well hidden in grain silos that olfaction is the only sense that can detect it. The wasp not only ferrets out its prey, but it can also tell by the scent what stage of development the prey has reached. A pupal caterpillar, which the wasp finds unsuitable, is never attacked.

At the opposite end of the scale are the animals that have little or no sense of smell. Many scientists maintain that most birds are in this category. The general truth of this claim is still under debate, but in many birds it has been established beyond doubt. The vultures are a good example: although the carrion these birds seek emits a putrid smell, they cannot find it if it is covered by a piece of cloth.

Vultures are sight-guided creatures in the truest sense of the term. They perch on any tall point found in their natural habitat, in treetops, on crags, and so on. When one of them notices carrion lying near by, it swoops down; other vultures notice the flight and follow, and they in turn are followed by still others perched farther away, so that dozens will congregate about the food in a matter of minutes.

Odorous substances

Sounds and colors can be classified in definite order, but smells seem to show a bewildering diversity. Cer-

tain scientists—among them the pioneer Carolus Lin-
naeus—have ventured the daring hypothesis that some
sort of system could also be established for smells. Lin-
naeus was followed by Zwaardemaker, who grouped
smells in nine different classes, and later by Hans Hen-
ning, who postulated the existence of only six classes—
spicy, flowery, fruity, resinous, putrid, and burnt. But
so far none of these attempts has shown any positive
results.

First of all, we have not yet established any clear link
between the sensation of smell and the substance which
causes it (the olficient). Here we become aware of the
enormous gap that exists between our fairly advanced
knowledge of optics and acoustics on the one hand and
our limited knowledge of olfaction on the other. Every
sound and color can be accurately linked with a certain
frequency of vibration or wave length, but no one knows
with any degree of certainty what distinguishes the various olficients from each other. To be sure, there is no
dearth of hypotheses in this difficult field, but in view of
their uncertainty we need not discuss them any further
here.

It used to be taken for granted that the volatility of the
olficients was their most important physical property, but
this theory was never proved. Some of the most potent
olficients, such as musk and vanillin, are not very volatile.
We know that the potent olficients are always highly
soluble in ether, whereas their solubility in water may
be extraordinarily low; but these properties have so far
been explored only from point of view of the human sense
of smell. We still know absolutely nothing about the
olficients that affect the olfactory sense of aquatic animals, such as the salamanders.

This last remark brings us to another field which is of
great significance for biology. Should we assume that
animals as different as mammals, fish, and insects react

to the same olfacients? We are still a long way from a general solution to this problem, but the most thorough investigation so far performed yielded a most unexpected answer. Karl von Frisch established through several long and careful tests that bees and human beings react to the same olfacients. Bees can be conditioned to react to any substance we can smell, but not to those which are odorless to us.

Students of the physiology of the senses find it particularly surprising that the number of possible olfactory sensations seems to be unlimited. There is a play in which a society lady unexpectedly lands in jail and makes the acquaintance of a number of human types she has never encountered before. She screams, "I have never known that there were such odors in the world!" This exclamation quite eloquently describes the situation. If we searched the entire world we would never find any really new sensations in the domains of color and of sound, but we must be prepared for anything where our noses are involved.

The chemical industry keeps turning out new products, many of which have smells that no human nose ever smelled before. This is the greatest of all the puzzles presented by our sense of smell. The layman may be inclined to see the logical answer in the theory that every new olfacient stimulates the nose in some totally new fashion. But we established in one of the preceding chapters that every sensory cell, regardless of how it is stimulated, always forwards the same excitation to the proper center. It scarcely seems reasonable to discard this universally accepted law.

Perhaps the only explanation which avoids these difficulties is the so-called theory of components. This theory assumes that the human nose houses a great number of different olfactory cells, each of which, when individually stimulated, produces a special sensation in the brain. It is extremely rare, however, that only one sort of cell is stimulated; even simple stimulants, such as ammonia, act on a number of cells. The resultant sensation is the product of the blending of all these primary sensations into a more complex one, just as an image is a completely homogeneous sensation, despite the fact that it is composed of innumerable visual impressions. If one smells an entirely new substance, such as osmic acid (OsO_4), it may stimulate a combination of sensory cells which have never before acted in concert; so a new olfactory image (if I may coin this rather daring term), and thus an entirely new sensation, has been created.

This theory is given some support by the fact that the smell of many olficients varies drastically according to their concentration. When ionone is strongly diluted it has the smell of violets, but in a certain concentration it smells like cedarwood. In order to understand this phenomenon, you need only imagine that different concentrations stimulate different sensory cells according to their specific threshold values. The combination of the sensory cells involved in the creation of the olfactory image—and thus the smell—varies with the concentration.

The sense of taste

In everyday life, people pay little notice to the function of the sense of taste. A well-prepared dinner means to the gourmet a great many exquisite dishes, each of them different from the others. But when you have a cold, you find that even the finest food gives you no pleasure and everything has a disgustingly flat taste, as though you were eating wood or straw. Thus we learn by personal experience that man actually tastes with his nose, and not with his tongue at all. Exquisite as a fine steak may taste, your tongue's sole contribution to your pleasure is the salty sensation. Delightful aromatic odors are released in your mouth as you chew the meat, and these odors ascend through the narrow nasopharyngeal opening to your nose; there, in the hidden folds of the olfactory epithelium, lie the real critics whose judgment will decide whether you praise or censure the cook. They notice if the stew is burnt or the butter rancid; they judge the quality of a new vintage.

The human tongue is clumsy in matters of taste; its language is limited to four words: sweet, sour, salty, bitter. Anatomists tell us that only certain parts of the tongue are sensitive to taste stimuli; these spots, chiefly in the back and on the edges, are equipped with taste buds, which are simple groups of a few sensory cells (Fig. 43). Many of these buds respond only to one of the four types of taste, others to two, still others to three or to all four of them.

The sources of these four varieties of taste vary widely. For humans, the salty taste can be traced to only one substance, ordinary table salt, which is common in nature. All other salts are in addition either sour or bitter. The sour taste is produced only by a few acids—or, to use the current scientific term, by free H-ions. The situation is different with respect to the other two tastes, sweet and bitter. Neither of these is specific to any particular group of substances. Certain elements, such

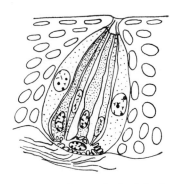

FIG. 43. A taste bud of the human tongue.

as magnesium, taste bitter, but so do various quite simple nitro-compounds, as well as such highly complex chemical compounds as quinine.

Sweetness we know chiefly from our experience with certain sugars, yet saccharine, a synthetic substance which has no chemical affinity with any sugar, also tastes sweet. A great deal of ingenuity has been expended on attempts to demonstrate what these substances have in common, but all such efforts have failed to produce any tangible result—presumably because the question was improperly formulated. We have found that the sensations do not originate in the sensory cells, but in the brain. We might say, therefore, that "sweet" is the taste sensation produced by the stimulation of those taste cells whose nerve tracks run to the sensory center for sweetness. Since different kinds of these taste cells react to different substances, a wide variety of substances may very well have the same taste.

The decisive factor is not the chemical constitution of the substances tasted, but the structure of our sensory apparatus. Both "sweet" and "bitter" have a broad biological significance. The sweet taste, always linked with a pleasurable sensation, serves to attract the animal to a source of nourishment that is both pleasing and beneficial to it. The bitter taste, on the other hand, is a danger signal. By studying our use of language we can see how fundamental this evaluation is. Everything that generates joy is called sweet: love, sleep, a child, or a beautiful woman; while anything unpleasant, such as death or pain, is decried as bitter.

In the study of the sense of taste in animals, the first question has usually been to what extent it is like our own. But despite the fundamental similarity, there are all sorts of differences. The cat, for instance, is not acquainted with the sensation we know as "sweet," and the dog does not react to saccharine. Many vertebrates, especially birds, show little sensitivity to bitter substances; birds often like to eat bitter seeds. This sense seems to be absent in the amphibians as well. Toads have been observed to swallow with gusto meal worms soaked in quinine.

A big surprise to scientists was the evidence that fish have a much finer sense of taste than the rest of the vertebrates. This characteristic is probably linked with the fact that in fish there is still no connection between the oral cavity and the nose, so that the sense of taste must do its own work. A minnow is 500 times more sensitive to sugar than we humans, and 184 times more sensitive than we are to table salt.

Some insects are amazingly sensitive to taste. We already know that many butterflies and flies are equipped with taste cells not merely on their mouth parts, but on their forelegs as well. As a result, the differences in sensitivity are still greater here. For instance, an admiral, a common multicolored butterfly, reacts to a 0.003 per cent solution of raw sugar, whereas 0.4 per cent is the minimum to which a human responds.

6. The Sense of Touch

The accomplishments of the human sense of touch

A man coming home late at night feels his way cautiously along the long dark hallway, trying not to wake the other people in the house, until he finally manages to slip into his own room. Here is an example of the primary purpose of the sense of touch: to keep us from bumping into hard objects while finding our way about without the use of our other senses. Although civilized people seldom find themselves in such situations, the sense of touch is nevertheless an important and indispensable friend to animals in their natural habitat.

Just as an army sends out advance scouts, many organisms have developed special organs of touch—such as antennae and tactile hairs—which reconnoiter the terrain in advance of the rest of the organism. In most animals, the rest of the body is also sensitive to touch. Scattered over the skin of a human, for instance, are spots of delicate subcutaneous sensory nerve endings. You can find them by touching various parts of your skin with a hair. Each person has an estimated total of 640,000 such tactile areas, but they are not equally thick in all parts of the body. In some places, notably on the hands and on the face, they are clustered densely together, whereas on the back they are more widely spaced. All these areas are so minute that a person usually has the illusion that the entire surface of his body is uniformly sensitive to touch.

Man's hand has developed far beyond its original use, and has become his most sensitive organ of touch, conveying to him much important information. The sensitivity of the hand is doubtless due to the extraordinary density of its tactile areas. Because of this density, an excitation rarely affects a single pressure point; a large number of them are usually affected simultaneously.

The time element, too, is often important when one is trying to determine the nature and properties of an object. As you run your hand over the surface of an object, the number of tactile areas consecutively exposed to different stimuli will tell you whether the object is rough or smooth or sticky. In some cases, however, you can gain a distinct impression without moving your hand. When you lay your hand on a straw mat, the different sensations experienced by the tactile elements allow you to conclude that the mat is rough.

The sense of touch conveys a distinct idea of the location of objects in space; thus it is capable, although to a lesser extent, of a function similar to that of the eye. The human skin can even be used for reading. With your fingers, write a numeral on someone's back; he will be able to tell with a considerable degree of accuracy what number it is.

Man's sensitivity to touch has made possible the construction of an alphabet for the blind (Fig. 44). The Braille alphabet is certainly one of the most beneficial inventions of man, for it has enabled thousands of people who were deprived of their eyesight to share, unaided, the written cultural heritage of mankind. The alphabet was named for its inventor, the Frenchman Louis Braille (1809–1852); it consists of letters based on a system of six dots arranged in two vertical columns. For each letter symbol some combination of dots is raised above the surface, so that a blind person can feel them with his fingertips. "Reading" a Braille text requires only three or four times as long as ordinary visual reading.

Another astonishing accomplishment of the blind is their possession of a "sixth sense," a space sense which makes them aware of the presence of solid objects without physical contact. It should hardly be necessary to mention that this is no special attribute of the blind alone; every human being has the sense, but few exercise it. As you walk through a dark hallway, you find that you are suddenly aware of where the hallway ends, even without touching the wall. Just how one develops this awareness has never been scientifically explained. Air currents, which are reflected by all solid objects, certainly play some part in it, and the heat sense may be involved, since the temperature of a solid is often slightly different from that of the surrounding air. But the whole answer is yet to be found.

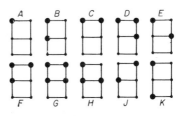

FIG. 44. The letters *A* to *K* of the Braille alphabet.

When you are pricked, pinched, or pushed, you are aware not only of what happened but also of where it happened. From this fact we know that within the brain there are innumerable tactile representatives, each connected with the tactile cells of different areas of the body. The high precision which this localization has attained can be convincingly demonstrated by a neat little experiment. Take a ball about half an inch in diameter (a child's marble will do best) and roll it back and forth on the table between the tips of the index and middle fingers of one hand. Your impression will be simply that you are touching a spherical object. Now cross your index and middle fingers and roll the same ball between their tips. Because of the unusual position of your fingertips you will experience an amazing sensory illusion: you will have the distinct impression that you are handling two separate balls. A person who tried this experiment for the first time with his eyes closed would swear that there were two marbles between his fingertips. What is the explanation of this illusion? The adjacent halves of any two neighboring fingers—the right side of the right index finger and the left side of the right middle finger—send their perceptions to the same center. If, however, the same two fingers are crossed, the sphere will touch the other half of each—in this case the left side of the right index finger and the right side of the right middle finger —and those halves report their impressions to two different centers. The left side of the right index finger will now signal that it is touching a spherical object. The same signal will be forwarded by the right side of the right middle finger. Since the two signals are sent to different centers, the sensory image of two distinct balls is the result.

The tactile reflexes of animals

Whether you stand, sit, or lie down, some part of your body is always in contact with the surface beneath you.

Since you have grown accustomed to the pressure of the weight of your body on your feet, you are unpleasantly surprised when a rapidly descending elevator frees you temporarily of this pressure.

In the lower animals these tactile stimuli, which normally issue from the surfaces of the feet in contact with the soil, are most important. Everybody has seen a beetle lying on its back and kicking furiously with its six legs until it succeeds in getting back onto its feet. The beetle struggles so violently not because of its unaccustomed position but because it cannot bear to swing its feet around without touching anything. Its aim is to bring its feet into contact with a solid object again, and it will stop kicking instantly if you offer it a twig to grab.

An insect can let its legs dangle free only when it is flying. In fact, when in the air an insect feels a compulsion not to let its feet touch anything solid. A few insects that must carry things to their nests have managed to throw off this compulsion, but most insects are incapable of grabbing something with their feet and flying away with it. An ordinary fly, for instance, cannot carry anything through the air. If you want to investigate this statement, catch a fly and carefully glue its back to a piece of wire. It will soon begin to "fly," without changing its location in the slightest. If you observe closely you will notice that the fly holds its feet in the proper flight position: the front feet are extended forward, the hind ones backward, and the middle ones more or less at right angles to its body. If you take a tiny piece of paper, roll it up into a ball, and hold it between the fly's legs, the fly will cease its flying motions and "run around" on the ball, rolling it rapidly backward. The fly does not care whether it is moving relative to the ball, or the ball relative to it; since it is in contact with something, the fly feels thoroughly at ease. Unlike human beings, it needs no awareness of the pull of gravity; the sensation of having its feet touch a solid body is enough.

Leeches also demonstrate clearly the effect of tactile stimuli on the movements of an animal. A leech will either walk (alternately anchoring and releasing its front and rear suckers) or swim, depending on the sensations received by its tactile organs. When neither of its suckers has a hold on anything—for instance, if you tear it away from the object to which it is fastened and throw it into the water—it will swim. But swimming becomes impossible as soon as you allow its rear sucker to touch a solid object—even one as small as a tiny splinter of glass. If you then throw it into the water, it is as incapable of swimming as if it had never been in water. The tactile stimuli generated by the tiny mote of glass prevent the leech from executing any normal swimming movement, and it sinks sluggishly to the bottom.

If a cat falls from a roof, it will land feet first. Many bugs and other insects which cavort on the branches of trees can do the same trick. The source of this ability is the sense of touch: as soon as the feet of an insect lose contact with something solid, the absence of the accustomed tactile sensations on their feet stimulates a reflex action, the so-called flight posture, in which the back is arched backward and all six legs are held stiff, pointing as sharply backward as possible. The insect thus turns itself into a veritable parachute and without any special exertion lands with its underside toward the ground (Fig. 45).

In most animals the sense of touch becomes active only upon direct contact; in other words, their tactile range does not extend beyond their bodies. Some aquatic animals, however, possess what may well be called a long-range tactile sense. The organ which serves this sense is the lateral line system which is found in fish and some amphibians. It enables the animal not only to detect anything that moves in its vicinity, but even to

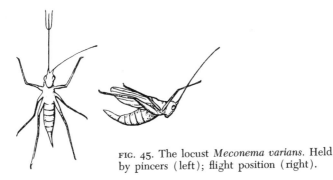

FIG. 45. The locust *Meconema varians*. Held by pincers (left); flight position (right).

determine its exact location. If you put a frog, *Xenopus laevis*, in an aquarium, lower a tiny ball on a thin wire into the water, and then make the ball swing gently back and forth about four inches behind the frog, where he cannot see it, the animal will turn at once and snap at the ball with its mouth. This is, of course, the method it uses to capture small animals which move in its proximity.

The muscular sense

This sense does not have a colloquial name; in fact most people have no idea of what it is. Yet, we use the muscular sense every day, on the most diverse occasions. It is, in short, the sense that sees to it that we use our muscles intelligently, to the exact extent required by the action to be performed. Evidence of the importance of this sense is given by the frequent occurrence in daily speech of such adjectives as *heavy, light, soft, hard, gaseous, liquid,* and *solid.*

Even a child knows that there are heavy and light objects, and that the criterion of "heavy" is the effort which it costs you to lift a specific object. It is obvious that we perceive heaviness—but *how* do we perceive it? We notice the pressure of contact exerted by the object on our hand as we lift it, but this does not completely account for the sensation. The elements mainly responsible for the sensation are the receptors of the muscular sense, the muscular spindles, located in both the muscles and tendons.

Let us see how this sense functions. Before a shot-putter hurls the iron ball, he first tests its weight by swinging it back and forth. As he does so, the weight of the ball is impressed upon his muscular sense, and he will gauge the force of his thrust according to the reports which the muscular sense sends to his brain. It has been determined that by means of this sense a human being can distinguish between a weight of 800 grams and one of 804 grams (28.22 and 28.36 oz.).

"Soft" and "hard" seem at first to be perceptions derived from tactile sensations, but the muscular sense has at least an equal share in their formulation. We judge whether an object is hard or soft by the resistance it offers to an attempt to change its shape. A hard object first produces a deformation in the fleshy part of the finger; as we press our examination, however, bone and muscle are brought into play, and we appraise the degree of its hardness by the resistance we encounter. The same method of appraisal is the basis of the concepts "liquid" and "solid." A "liquid" is something which, though we can feel it, offers no resistance to an attempt to penetrate it. "Gaseous" is a designation applied to a body that affects neither our sense of touch nor our muscular sense.

The muscular sense can be demonstrated in forms of life as low on the evolutionary scale as the worms. If you offer a leech some object to which it can attach its front sucker, it contracts its body so as to make it as short as possible, and it is able then to support a heavy weight placed on its hind sucker. In this position the leech can hold up thirty times its own weight for several minutes. If you support the weight with your hand for a moment, the leech's muscular sense instantly informs it of this change, and it adjusts its muscles to the lighter weight. The result is that as soon as you withdraw your hand, the return of the unaccustomed weight stretches out the body of the leech.

7. *The Heat Sense*

In the searing rays of the summer sun, a dog will stretch out lazily on the sand and show in every possible manner his complete satisfaction with life. His behavior demonstrates that one of the most important functions of the heat sense is to make the animal seek out the places where the temperature is most pleasant. The lizards, cold-blooded creatures who bask on burning hot rocks, and the big bluebottle flies who perch on sun-baked walls, are guided by the pleasant sensation of warmth.

Favorable temperature

In our latitudes the temperature is unlikely to rise too high for any animal. It is easy, however, to demonstrate by experiments that for every creature there is a favorable temperature. The extremely simple and practical instrument invented for this purpose is called a "temperature organ." It is a long, narrow box with a lighted gas burner under one end and ice cooling the other end, so that a temperature drop occurs from one end to the other. If you put in the box a considerable number of animals of any one species—let us say, a hundred ants—you will find that very soon most of them congregate within a relatively narrow strip, the area of their favorable temperature.

These animals have, of course, no inkling of what they accomplish by seeking out that particular temperature, the optimal one for their organisms. The warmth to which they expose themselves does not limit itself to satisfying the sensory cells; it pervades the entire body of the animal. In a cold-blooded creature it causes every function—breathing, digestion, and so on—to run its course much more rapidly and energetically than it could at a lower temperature. The utilization of the heat of the sun is of great importance to many animals, especially in the cool spring season. In many cases the effect of a difference in temperature acquires an additional significance. All the insect pests which plague man and feed on him—bedbugs, lice, gadflies, and the like—are stimulated by heat to move toward its source in order to find their prey.

We know relatively little about the anatomy of the temperature sense, even in man. It probably has no sensory cells at all in the skin. Fine nerve endings in the skin, whose cell bodies are situated only in the spinal cord, serve as the end organs. You can locate them by exploring your skin with the aid of a hot or cold needle; as you do so, you will discover two remarkable facts. The first is that we are dealing with two distinct senses: a heat sense and a cold sense. An individual point that is sensitive to heat can never perceive cold, and a point sensitive to cold is likewise unable to register heat. The second fact is that the sensation of heat or cold has absolutely nothing to do with pain. Daily experience seems to teach that these two sensations blend into each other. If you touch an object whose temperature is rising, your sensation seems to change from warmth through heat to pain. This is, however, an illusion. If you heat an individual heat-sensitive point in the same fashion, you will never sense pain, for the pain occurs only when the heat excites the adjacent sensory endings of the pain sense.

A further peculiarity of our heat sense is the great difference in the sensitivity of the various parts of the body. For the sense of touch, the most exposed parts of the body, such as the hands and the feet, are the most highly sensitive, but for the heat sense the situation is the contrary. The middle parts of the body—the back or the buttocks—respond most readily to temperature stimuli. Biologically, this suggests that the heat sense watches over the temperature conditions of the entire body. To the body as a whole it means little if the hands freeze, but if the torso is cold, the situation will probably manifest itself throughout the body by a lowering of the temperature of the blood. These temperature-sensitive spots must therefore send alarm signals to the body in time. Another interesting aspect of the regulation of temperature is the fact that the cold sense is far more widespread over the body than the heat sense. This situation is also easy to explain: man, having lost the natural hairy covering of the mammals, finds cold a far more ominous stimulus than heat.

The regulation of body heat

The search for the most favorable exterior temperature is of less importance to warm-blooded than to cold-blooded creatures. The warm-blooded animals differ from all other forms of animal life in that they have to a great extent emancipated themselves from the effects of changes in external conditions. They have as a result populated the earth in every latitude from the icy North Pole to the even icier South Pole, and in all elevations from the sea shores to the eternally snow-capped mountain peaks. The freedom of these animals stems primarily from their ability to keep their body heat at a constant level under any climatic conditions.

We human beings regulate our body heat first of all with our clothing. Common phrases such as "not smart enough to keep warm" show that we recognize the fact that keeping warm does, after all, require a little intelligence. Animals, short on the ability to reason, keep warm by reflex action—and with greater efficiency. When a human being or an animal begins to feel too hot, all the valves of the body open up to permit the heat to escape. Dilatation of fine capillaries in the skin serves this purpose. In a human being this takes place in the face, and in a rabbit over the entire surface of the long ears, which are spread out from the body. When the African sun beats down, the elephant uses its gigantic ears as heat equalizers in the same way; it also uses them to fan itself, and their movement permits surplus heat to escape from its body. Horses and many other animals discharge perspiration all over their bodies; the cooling effect is produced by the slow evaporation of the perspiration from the skin. When a dog feels too hot, it lets its wet tongue loll out and draws cool air into its lungs in short, rapid breaths.

When it gets too cold, other body mechanisms become active. As you emerge blue with cold after your first outdoor swim of the season, you shiver like a bowl of jelly. Animals shiver too—witness the phrase, "shivering like a young pup." The layman is accustomed to regarding this phenomenon as a highly undesirable accompaniment of the sensation of cold, but in reality it is of great practical value. Cold excites the muscles to this reflex action, which is their way of producing a considerable amount of heat to counteract the drop in temperature. In addition the cutaneous capillaries, which open up when it is hot, contract in the cold—thus retaining the heat. Cold also intensifies the metabolic processes, so as to generate more heat.

In mammals and birds these heat-regulating processes are not due exclusively to excitation of the sensory cells of the skin. The blood carries the heat to the brain, where certain centers contain heat-sensitive cells. The excitation of these cells sets off the regulating processes. Thus, despite the fact that there are no temperature-sensitive cells in the skin, heat regulation is nevertheless to be considered a genuine sensory function.

Scientists used to believe that the cold-blooded lower forms of animal life had nothing like the highly intricate regulatory mechanisms of the higher forms; this conceit is gradually being exploded. The beekeepers learned a long time ago that it never got very cold in a beehive, but nobody knew why. Then a German bee breeder decided to take readings of the temperature in several beehives every few hours, day and night, throughout an entire winter. His observations were later rechecked with the aid of intricate scientific apparatus which automatically recorded the readings, and his findings were confirmed. The temperature in the beehives fluctuated constantly, yet never dropped below a certain minimum.

The explanation is remarkable. In the winter, tens of thousands of bees in a hive cluster closely together. The bees in the center of the cluster are warm enough when the temperature drops, but those in the outer layers get cold; they then begin to kick their feet and flap their wings rapidly—in other words, they act much as we do when we shiver with the cold. The main thing seems to be, though, that their agitation spreads through the entire cluster of 10,000 or more bees. The concerted efforts of the group eventually generates a sizable amount of heat. The temperature consequently rises until all the bees have calmed down, and then gradually drops until the same process is repeated.

Heat regulation can be observed in other social insects during the summer. For instance, the red forest ants (*Formica rufa*) in their big dome-shaped nests know how to generate a temperature of about 74 to 84 degrees Fahrenheit, the most favorable temperature range for their young. When the sun shines, the ants make numerous holes in the dome to let the heat in; these holes are closed again at sundown. The opposite problem faces the small wasps, *Polistes gallica,* who fasten their nests to rocks and must protect them from becoming overheated. This they accomplish by carrying in droplets of water which they fan with their wings until the water evaporates.

Perhaps even more surprising is the fact that the moths, which lead solitary lives, also possess a heat regulator of a sort. Every youngster who has indulged in the pastime of collecting butterflies must have observed that the thick-bodied sphinx, bombycid, and noctuid moths go through a peculiar maneuver before taking off on their nocturnal flights: they make their wings whir so rapidly that they seem almost invisible to an observer only a few inches away. They keep up this effort for several minutes, then all of a sudden they spread their wings and vanish. It took natural scientists a long time to discover what was behind this behavior. They knew very well that it had to have some significance, because such a moth cannot fly unless he has gone through this preflight ritual. If you pick one up before he has fluttered his wings, and release him, he will plummet to the ground like a stone. We can guess the answer: this is another version of the peculiar shivering movements we have observed in mammals and in bees exposed to cold. Here, too, heat is generated through the quivering of the strong flying muscles, and the flight cannot commence until an adequate amount of heat has been generated. When such insects are kept in a cage at a constant 86 degrees Fahrenheit, they will take off immediately after being released. In this case, too, we can understand how the heat is regulated only if we assume that the heat is perceived by the sensory apparatus of the moth, even though we have no idea where the heat-sensitive cells are located.

8. *Gravity*

Life blankets our earth like a thin crust, as the thin surface layer of wax covers a plum. Life penetrates the surface of the earth no deeper than the nethermost roots of the trees, nor does it reach higher than the lowest layers of the atmosphere. As the oceans are populated most densely in their upper strata, we see that most life thrives on the border between the air above and the earth and water below. The factor that determines this habitable area is, of course, the force of gravity, which for this and other reasons is of immeasurable importance in the shaping of life.

As long as an organism moves in a horizontal plane, it will encounter the same conditions of life everywhere. But when it moves in a vertical direction, climbing a mountain or diving down into the murky depths of the sea, it will encounter a change in practically all the factors on which life depends—temperature, atmospheric pressure, light, and so forth. It is thus a matter of paramount importance for every form of life to control the direction of its motion. This is particularly true of creatures that move freely in their natural element, such as the fish and the birds. Fish mostly swim in a horizontal plane, but they must also be capable of swimming straight up or straight down if need be. For this purpose they are equipped with sense organs that inform them of the direction of the force of gravity.

Scientists are handicapped in the investigation of these sense organs by the fact that the excitation of the organ does not produce any sensation, but expresses itself in involuntary movements. Such movements can be studied much better in animals, which—unlike a human being— can be interrogated with a knife instead of a questionnaire. If we were forced to depend on human beings, we would still have very little information about these things. But the small invertebrates, because of the extremely clear and easily comprehensible structure of their gravity-sensitive organs, have contributed a great deal to the solution of the entire problem. Let us therefore start our survey with these creatures, first taking a look at an organ known as a statocyst.

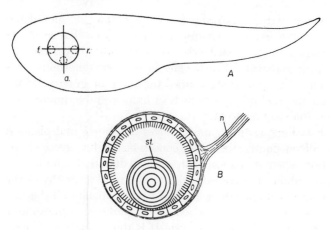

FIG. 46. *A*, diagrammatic sketch of an animal with statocyst; *B*, the statocyst itself. *f.*, front pole; *r.*, rear pole; *a.*, abdominal pole; *st.*, statolith; *n.*, nerve.

The statocyst and its reflexes

A statocyst has all the features of a well-designed mechanical device, for it is extremely simple and yet consummately practical. In its simplest form the statocyst is a liquid-filled sphere whose inner wall is almost completely lined with sensory cells. In addition to the liquid, the sphere also contains a round stone, the statolith; since the statolith consists mostly of calcareous matter which is heavier than the liquid, it always rolls to the lowest point of the spherical sac. The statocyst is designed to keep the animal informed at all times of the direction of the force of gravity. To determine that direction, we simply draw a line connecting the center of the sac and the point where the statolith touches the wall.

In all vertebrates, including man, the simple spherical statocyst has developed into a very intricate apparatus, the labyrinth. It contains, first of all, two irregular cavities, the utricle and the saccule, with typical statoliths inside them. Each cavity is the site of a special sense organ: the saccule is the home of the organ of hearing, the cochlea, and the utricle houses the three semicircular canals which we shall discuss a little later.

The statocyst, like the globe, can be assigned a number of cardinal points relative to the body that contains it: the front pole, the rear pole, the abdominal pole, and so on. If the animal wants to swim straight up, it assumes a position in which the statolith touches the rear pole of the sac (Fig. 46). If the animal retains this position while swimming, it is a mathematical certainty that it will move straight up. To swim straight down, it must turn its body until the statolith touches the front pole of the sensory sac; if it wants to swim horizontally, the abdominal pole must receive the pressure of the statolith.

The statocyst and the labyrinth also help swimming and flying animals to maintain their balance. Every animal that moves about freely in its natural element keeps both sides of its body level. How does it do this? When the animal is level, the statolith will touch a certain point on each side of the sac wall. If the animal gets off balance, the touch of the stone stimulates an immediate compensatory movement of the sensory epithelium, which

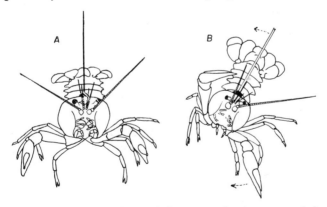

FIG. 47. Equilibrium reflexes of the river crab. *A*, posture of the normal animal in a vertical position; *B*, in a slanted position with the legs on the lower-situated side steering. (After Kühn.)

restores the body to its normal level position (Fig. 47).

It would be a mistake to believe that the animal consciously controls these movements—that when the statolith lies in an unusual position the creature realizes something is wrong and turns its body until it can say, "This is it! The stone lies right now, so I must be swimming horizontally." Inasmuch as conscious sensations of this nature are absent even in human beings, they must certainly be absent in fish, crayfish, or squids. The process is a series of unconscious reflex movements.

A fish is struck by a powerful wave and hurled on its side. When such an accident occurs, the fish does not have to think about its position very long; whether it likes it or not, the statoliths in its utricle change their position and press against a new set of sensory hairs. These excited sensory cells, normally not accustomed to excitation, send forth signals that excite the motor nerves leading to the muscles of its body and fins. The fins immediately shift into a slanting position, one stretching out stiffly, the other one flattening down, and the fish turns back into its accustomed upright position.

The explanation that the organism is made aware of gravity by the pressure of a tiny pebble on a few minute sensory hairs struck many natural scientists as too simple to be true.

Since there are several organisms that can orient themselves quite efficiently without any such apparatus, all sorts of other hypotheses were offered. Finally, a brilliant idea of the Austrian scientist Kreidl removed the statolith question from the raging tempest of theories onto the solid ground of fact. The order Decapoda of the class Crustacea (the order of the crustaceans equipped with five pairs of walking legs) includes not only the clumsy, sluggish lobsters and crayfish, but also the agile shrimps and prawns. In all these animals, the statocysts are situated at the base of the first pair of antennules (feelers) and communicate with the outside through fine, slotlike openings. The statoliths do not form and grow in the interior of the statocyst chamber, but are foreign bodies, such as grains of sand, which the animal itself inserts into the slot with its fine claws. Since each time it molts the creature sheds the entire statolith mass along with its outer covering, it has to replace the statolith at intervals.

Kreidl hit on the lucky idea of removing all the sand from the aquarium in which he kept his shrimps; just as the shrimps were about to molt, the sand was replaced by iron filings. The animals had no choice but to put the filings into their statocysts. Now, iron filings are strongly affected by magnets. Just imagine how Kreidl's shrimps must have felt when he held a magnet over them. The iron statoliths immediately hurtled against the sensory hairs on the upper wall of the sensory sac—precisely the position they occupy in a normal shrimp that has flopped on its back. The shrimp responded by turning over, and the statolith hypothesis was upheld.

When a fish is flung on its side, its eyes try to compensate for the change in position. Take a goldfish—whose eyes are directed outward almost at right angles to the body—and turn it on its left side. If you look at the fish from the rear, you will notice that its eyes no longer look out at right angles; the right eye, which is the upper one now, stares toward the abdominal side, while the left one has turned toward its back—you can distinctly make out the big, black pupil (Fig. 48). As long

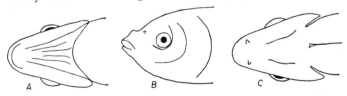

FIG. 48. The positional reflex of the eyes of a goldfish. *A*, the goldfish lying on its right side, viewed from its underside; *B*, in its normal position; *C*, lying on its left side, viewed from the back. (Original.)

as you keep the fish in this position, its eyes maintain these directions. So close is the link between the sense of position and the sense of vision, whenever the fish changes its position its eyes automatically make counter-movements to keep their original visual fields. The same thing takes place in a human being, but by optical means.

Let us return for a moment to the forms of life highest on the evolutionary scale, the mammals and man. We have inherited our entire intricate sensory apparatus from our remote ichthyoid (fishlike) ancestors. The eye and the labyrinth were originally designed for the ichthyoids —for their way of life, not ours. The transition to life on land brought many changes in both these senses. Man has lost a great many of the labyrinthian reflexes that function with such a high degree of precision in the fish. Great changes have also taken place in the other mammals.

While the head of a fish is joined directly to its body as rigidly as possible, the head of a mammal is linked to its body by the neck, with as much flexibility as possible. It is obviously important for a dog to be able to turn his head freely in all directions. One moment he is sniffing at the ground, the next he holds his muzzle high to catch some scent borne by the breeze, and a second

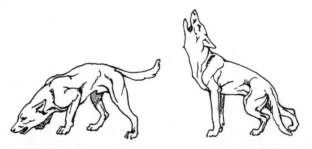

FIG. 49. A dog in two different postures, demonstrating the dependence of the position of the limbs on that of the head and neck.

later he uses it to hunt for a bothersome flea that is having a meal somewhere on his body. If the head performs all these diverse movements efficiently, it cannot be concerned about the labyrinth which it houses. Although the fish's labyrinth requires that the fish assume a certain normal position, this is not true of most mammals. Instead, a whole group of peculiar reflexes have made their appearance between the head and the neck and between the head and the legs. When the head (and with it the labyrinth) changes position, there ensues, unknown to the animal, a change in the extensor tonus, the muscular force that extends the legs. This tonus is weak when the muzzle hangs low and the neck is held high, and strong when the muzzle is higher than the neck.

The biological significance of these reflexes can be readily recognized. When a cat or a dog wants to reach something with its muzzle, a movement of its head and neck alone is usually not sufficient. A dog cannot eat from a dish on the floor unless it bends its forelegs and lowers its head and neck at the same time. If it held its forelegs straight, it would never be able to reach the food in the dish, because its neck is too short (Fig. 49). It is commonly believed that the dog assumes this well-known "drinking posture" by conscious, voluntary action; this notion, however, is wrong. Simple co-ordinations like this one are reflexes. Nature constantly tries to relieve the volition of all tasks in order to save it for use as a last resort.

How the cat falls from the roof

Cats, rabbits, dogs, monkeys, frogs, and many other animals can be dropped from a supine position without risk of injury. They know how to twist around in free fall with such speed that they land feet-first. This fact had been known for a long time before the invention of the motion-picture camera furnished science with a chance to analyze the movement. The first such study was inspired by the Paris Academy of Sciences in 1894. It established, first of all, that this maneuver was not a planned acrobatic feat like the death-defying leap of a circus performer, but a case of precise orientation in space. A trapeze artist in the circus gives himself an impetus so calculated as to make him twist about in mid-air exactly once before he lands. To execute this feat, he must know the exact height of his fall. But when cats were dropped into a pitch-dark shaft whose depth they did not know, they invariably landed on their feet regardless of the height from which they fell.

An acrobat pushes with his legs against the ground to give himself an initial impetus. A cat does not require this: if you suspend a cat upside down from several strings and suddenly cut all the strings at the same time, the animal will still land feet-first. It must therefore twist its body around while it falls. It has been proved, furthermore, that the labyrinth is necessary for this mid-air twist. Cats with both labyrinths removed plummet to the ground like so many bags of cement and land in any position. As soon as a normal cat loses its support the so-called head-positioning reflex occurs, bringing the head into its normal upright position. This movement naturally distorts the position of the neck, for the body is still in its original supine position. The neck-positioning reflex occurs next: the neck and subsequently the thorax follow the head and assume their proper positions. Finally, the hind section of the body follows suit. The twist thus takes place as a very rapid spiral movement of the entire body beginning with the head.

If this were all the cat did, however, it would never land on its feet. There is a law of physics which stipulates that an unattached or unsupported body will retain its position in space. If you climb up a rope, holding on with your hands and feet, then suddenly let go with your right hand and swing your right arm to the right,

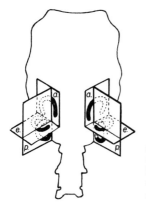

FIG. 50. Spatial position of the semi-circular canals of a pigeon. The skull is shown viewed from the rear. *a.*, *canalis anterior; e., canalis externus; p., canalis posterior.* (After Ewald.)

your body will turn a proportionate distance to the left so that the *status quo* remains unchanged. In order to execute its twist in mid-air despite this law of physics, the cat must perform quite intricate movements with its front and hind legs. Although they have not yet been analyzed these movements have been photographed. A cat ought to study physics before taking such a risk. It can perform an act with reflexes which it could never accomplish by conscious volition, even if it concentrated all of its intelligence on the task.

The semicircular canals

The semicircular canals—which, as we have seen, exist only in the vertebrates—function on a principle entirely different from that of the utricle. The utricle responds to the force of gravity, but the semicircular canals would work even if gravity did not exist. Their purpose is not to bring the organism into a certain position relative to the earth, but to keep it in whatever position it occupies. Hence the semicircular canals not only support the statolithic organs in their function, but also amount to a technical improvement of the entire system.

The position of the three semicircular canals demonstrates most strikingly that they are concerned with orientation. The canals are arranged in three mutually perpendicular planes, representing the planes of space (Fig. 50). Despite this obvious connection, it took quite a long time to solve their riddle. The French scientist Pierre Flourens first called attention to the semicircular canals in 1824, but it was half a century later before Josef Breuer succeeded in developing a theory that explained their nature.

In order to understand how the semicircular canals work, let us pay an imaginary visit to a kindergarten. As we enter, we find several children busy sailing their toy boats in a tub. One boy's boat has sailed to the far side of the tub, out of reach; in order to bring it nearer, he quickly twists the tub halfway around. He accomplishes absolutely nothing by the maneuver. He has succeeded in twisting the tub around, but the water, because of its inertia, has retained its position relative to him and the tiny boat is still floating on the opposite side of the tub.

Now we shall do some experimenting with the tub. We cut a few pieces of black paper in the shape shown in Figure 51, and we fold them along the short dotted line. Then we paste their wide ends to the wall of the tub, making the narrow ends float in the water. We wait until the water has become still, and then we turn the tub with a sudden jerk either clockwise or counterclockwise (Fig. 51). Of course, our paper strips are de-

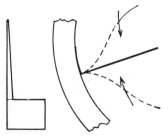

FIG. 51. Demonstration of the function of the semicircular canals. See text.

flected violently to one side. Since the tub was turned, but the water did not turn along with it, the water shifted its position relative to the tub, and the deflection of the strips of paper is the result of that relative shift.

This childish game has supplied us with a simple model of our semicircular canals. The end of each of them shows a small enlargement, like a tiny bulbous swelling, an ampulla. The entire canal is filled with a watery fluid. Every time you turn your head this fluid reacts exactly as did the water in the tub: it seeks, by its inertia, to retain its old position in space while the canal itself changes position, and so each turn of your head causes a deflection of the tuft of sensory hairs. This deflection is reported to your brain as a stimulus. Your brain then responds by a counterturn of your head which restores its old position in space. This is the principle on which the semicircular canals function.

9. *The Proprioceptive Sensory Elements*

Our senses are not by any means attuned exclusively to stimuli from the outside world. The body itself is a self-contained world, a microcosm, in which the proprioceptors (internal receptors for physical stimuli situated in the skin, the muscles, and the tendons) constantly send forth reports to the brain.

The posture sense

The best-known example is the posture sense. Just as a general must know the exact positions of his regiments and divisions in a battle in order to use them properly, so must the brain, the organ in command of the entire body, be kept accurately informed of what the individual limbs are doing and where they are. This is the faculty that enables you to tell accurately and instantly, even with your eyes closed, what position your arm or hand occupies, the way each individual finger is bent, the position of the wrist, and the angle of the elbow. When you reach out for some object, the required movements obviously depend not only on the location of that object, but on the initial position of your arm and hand as well. You owe the sureness of your reach to the fact that your brain is always aware of the position of your limbs and gauges the movement of the muscles accordingly.

The act of reaching for an object is more complicated than it might seem. An adult can touch the tip of his nose, his left ear, his right knee, or any other specific part of his body with absolute ease. This ability, so essential to normal life, is not come by without effort. We all spent countless hours of our earliest infancy in exploring our bodies by such movements of reaching and touching. It is by no means an easy job at first. The clumsy little hand of a baby does not know as yet how to shoo off a fly that has brazenly settled on his forehead. Sureness comes only gradually, increasing with practice and experience. The complications increase when you reach for a movable part of your body. If you want to touch your right knee, the action of your arm depends entirely on where your knee happens to be. These movements involve no difficulty for an adult. Your knee reports its momentary position to your brain through the sensory elements of the expandable skin of your thigh, and your brain determines from this report the nature and number of excitations that must be sent to the arm muscles to make the arm move in the proper fashion.

The judgment of distance

When some object attracts your attention, you turn your eyes so as to cause the image of the object to be projected exactly onto the *fovea centralis* of your retina, the spot on which the clearest images are perceived. In this process, each eye is moved by six muscles endowed

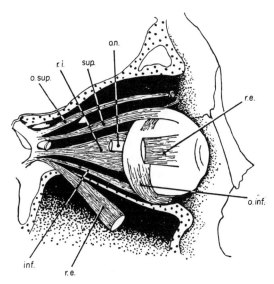

FIG. 52. The human eye and the ocular muscles. *o.n.*, optic nerve; *r.e.*, rectus exterior; *r.i.*, rectus interior; *sup.*, rectus superior; *inf.*, rectus inferior; *o. sup.*, obliquus superior; *o. inf.*, obliquus inferior.

with an extremely sensitive muscular sense (Fig. 52). The contraction of each muscle obviously depends not only on what part of the retina received the image first, but also on the position the eye occupied relative to the head at that instant.

Our ability to judge the distances between us and the objects about us is also dependent on the muscular sense. A one-eyed man will frequently pour the tea on the table before or behind his cup; he is severely handicapped in judging the location of the cup, since this judgment depends on the simultaneous action of both eyes. The simplest way to understand how this process works is to think of gunnery aboard a warship. The gunnery officer uses a range finder, a long tube with optical devices fastened to both ends. The distance of

the target and the elevation of the gun barrel are calculated from the angle formed by the axes of the two
instruments.

This is exactly what we do. Our range finders are our
eyes, which we train on the target by means of our six
pairs of ocular muscles. The distance is determined from
the angle formed by the axes of the two eyes. The brain,
however, cannot measure the angle directly, but judges
it by the contraction of the six muscles moving each
eye. The extent of the contractions is reported to the
brain by the mechanical sensory endings posted in the
ocular muscles or in their tendons. Every vertebrate that
has eyes capable of movement uses the same process.
Even the chameleon when it grabs a fly with a lightning-
quick flick of its tongue must first train both its eyes on
the moving target in order to have its ocular muscles
inform it of how far away the fly is.

Many acts require a combination of the muscular
sense of both the ocular muscles and the limbs. Most of
us are unaware of the complex processes involved in
hurling a stone at a target. Throwing stones at enemies
is no longer in vogue; but throughout the millennia that
preceded our modern civilization, expert marksmanship
with a stone was one of the most vital accomplishments
in life—as it certainly proved to be for David as he
felled Goliath. Perhaps this is the reason why the sensory
apparatus used in throwing is unbelievably intricate.

The eye guides and directs the throwing movement.
For this reason, a skilled pitcher or an expert pistol
marksman will snap his arm forward so that his hand
occupies a position right in the line of sight—so that the
target, his hand, and his sighting eye are in one straight
line. This is the secret of accurate marksmanship both
in shooting and in pitching. It is no more an innate
ability than is the ability to judge distances. A baby will
reach for the moon and must gain much experience before he realizes that such efforts are futile. The simple

art of judging distance is learned quite rapidly, however, while the complicated technique of pitching requires years of practice. It is understandable that even ten-year-olds are often quite clumsy when they try their hand at pitching.

We frequently combine the muscular sense with the sense of touch. It is not very difficult to determine the shape of an object in the dark. You run your hand along it and decide from the curved or angular movements of your hand whether the object it touches is spherical or cubical. You proceed in exactly the same fashion when you want to ascertain the size of an object by touch. In this case, your judgment is determined by the movement of your hand. In both cases, of course, your previous experience forms the basis for judgment.

Proprioceptors were believed for a long time to be a monopoly of the vertebrates. Today we know that these

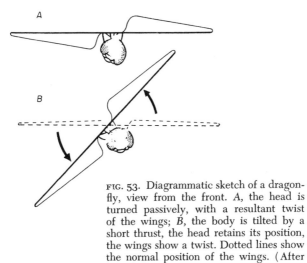

FIG. 53. Diagrammatic sketch of a dragon-fly, view from the front. A, the head is turned passively, with a resultant twist of the wings; B, the body is tilted by a short thrust, the head retains its position, the wings show a twist. Dotted lines show the normal position of the wings. (After Mittelstaedt.)

mechanisms are present in numerous invertebrates as well, and in all likelihood no form of animal life is without them. The use made of proprioceptors by the dragonflies is particularly interesting. These creatures are the most graceful aviators of all the insects in the world, the equal in flying skill of any bird. Unlike birds, however, dragonflies have no organ of equilibrium. They use their proprioceptors instead. The large head of the dragonfly, with its huge eyes, is joined to the body by an extremely slender neck. When a gust of wind tilts the body and the wings, the head's inertia keeps it in position (Fig. 53). The result is a twist in the neck and a consequent excitation of the proprioceptors situated on the back of the head. The wings are then shifted by a reflex movement that flashes out from these proprioceptors, and the normal position of the dragonfly is restored in a fraction of a second.

10. *The Combined Action of the Senses*

Wherever man may be, he is constantly exposed to many diverse stimuli which, in their varying combinations, constantly affect his inner life. The way these stimuli work together is therefore one of the most important questions of our sensory life. This relationship is as impossible to describe in one word as it would be to describe relationship of all the people we meet in life: in both cases there are friends and foes, as well as others whose spheres of activity never coincide. We must therefore take a number of different possibilities into account.

The double safety device

Every mechanic is familiar with the principle of the double safety device. When an engineer wants to ensure the proper operation of a piece of machinery under all possible circumstances, he installs two or more mutually independent devices; if one of them happens to break down, the remainder will guarantee the smooth operation of the unit. Nature developed this principle many millions of years before man discovered it. In order to ensure a biological action, nature frequently applies not just one but two or more stimuli. If some accident should prevent one stimulus from exerting its effect, the others guarantee the execution of the action. This concerted action of different senses is most dramatically manifested in the act of sexual intercourse, where the most various sensory stimuli guarantee a fertile union.

A far simpler case is the shrimp's device for maintaining its equilibrium (p. 140). When the shrimps are swimming in open waters, their statocysts compel them to keep their undersides toward the bottom of the sea. At the same time, they are also under a compulsion to turn their backs to the light. It is obvious that the stimulation from the light and the stimulation from the force of gravity have the same ultimate effect. The behavior of a shrimp will not be affected in the least if we block the light or if we remove its organs sensitive to the force of gravity, for its balance is doubly ensured.

This phenomenon should not be confused with the much rarer case in which the generation of an act requires two distinct stimuli. In this case, nothing happens when stimulus *A* occurs alone, nor when stimulus *B* occurs alone; the act will take place only if both *A* and *B* occur simultaneously. Let us illustrate this by an example. Between the spines on the hard shells of the sea urchins are remarkable pincer-like structures, pedicellariae. When this outer covering is stimulated, the tiny creatures react in an excited manner: they open their jaws, thrash about wildly, and they will seize and cling fast to anything that gets between their sharp-toothed jaws. The poisonous pedicellariae (Fig. 54) behave in a more reserved manner. They are the most important weapons the sea urchin has, and they are to be used only when an enemy, such as a starfish or some predatory snail, approaches. Now, the enemy is detected primarily

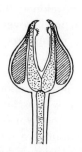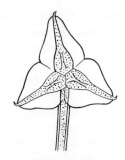

FIG. 54. Poison pedicellariae of a sea urchin. Closed (left); and opened (right).

by the sea urchin's chemical sense. The poisonous fluid, however, must not be discharged by the pedicellariae until the enemy is close enough to be grasped. For this reason, the pedicellariae are designed to react only when they are excited both chemically and mechanically at the same time, and this double stimulus occurs only when some part of the enemy's body gets between the saw-toothed jaws. This reaction can be studied in a most revealing experiment. If you excite the inner surfaces of the pincers by a mechanical stimulus—touching them with a fine bristle, for instance—they snap shut for an instant and then immediately open again. If you excite them only by a chemical stimulus (which never occurs in nature), the poison glands discharge their fluid, but the pincers do not close at all. But when both stimuli are applied simultaneously, the poison is discharged and the jaws snap firmly shut.

The cancellation of one stimulus by another

It frequently happens that two stimuli coincide, even though they were not meant to complement each other or to act in conjunction. When two such stimuli interfere with each other, one of them cancels out the other. A neat example is the scratch reflex in dogs. If you tickle the flank of a dog, it will raise a hind leg and scratch the spot. But if you tickle both its flanks at the same time, the dog cannot very well scratch both sides of its body simultaneously, for after all it needs its legs to stand on. As a result, there will be no response on the side of the weaker stimulation.

Cases of two stimuli competing for dominance occur quite frequently, if not in nature at least in controlled experiments. The classic example of such a dilemma is the famous parable of Buridan's ass, the animal which starved to death between two big stacks of hay because it was unable to choose between the two. To be sure, no mention of this ass occurs in the writings of Jean Buridan, a great French philosopher of the fourteenth century; his opponents originated the story in order to ridicule him. The truth is that there are very few such fools among the lower animals.

In order to demonstrate this to yourself, simply place two lights before a phototactic animal, thus forcing it to decide which way to move. Most insects and crustaceans (including the tiny water fleas), the starfish and several Chaetopoda will eventually make a decision and approach one of the two lights. It is quite amusing to watch the animal vacillate between the two stimuli, like a human being who is unable to make up his mind. The water flea will swim a short distance toward the light on its left, then will turn to the other; soon it changes its mind again, and so it keeps moving back and forth in a zigzag.

It sometimes happens that different stimuli directly interfere with each other. Let us take another look at the agile shrimps as they dart back and forth in the seaweed. As long as they keep swimming, they must obey their statocysts, which compel them to swim with their undersides facing the sea bottom. But as soon as the shrimps' slender legs touch an alga or a rock, they are no longer subject to this compulsion. If this were not the case, the compulsion would be an intolerable hardship, for it would not permit the animal to rest anywhere but on perfectly horizontal surfaces. Fortunately shrimps can settle down for a rest in any desired position without the least concern about gravity. This is due to the fact that the tactile stimuli which they receive through their feet nullify the gravitational stimuli. But let us remember that shrimps swimming free of contact with anything solid are compelled by their eyes to turn their backs toward the light. This is a form of negative phototropism, and it might well be named "photodorsal reflex." How is this reflex counteracted when a shrimp is in contact with a solid object? The ability of a shrimp to sit on a slope appears to prove that the sense of touch of its feet has an inhibitory effect on its eyes, too. But it is easy to demonstrate that this is not the case at all. If we remove the statocysts of the shrimp, it will shift immediately to a position called for by the photodorsal reflex, which has its first opportunity to manifest its effect unimpeded. Thus, there are three stimuli competing for supremacy. While the tactile impressions of the feet nullify the gravitational stimuli, the latter in turn impede the eyes from exercising their effect.

Freedom of the will

Philosophers deal with Man, whose complexity continually poses new questions. Biologists like to deal occasionally with quite simple forms of life, which in most cases give a simple answer to a simple question. In almost every instance, lower forms of animal life respond to a certain stimulus with a certain reaction, a compulsive action if you like, which is apt to make one speak, mistakenly, of a reflex. We have mentioned that if you shoo away a fly that disturbs your morning slumber, it will flee straight through the window to safety outside. But if you scare away a cat that has sneaked in through a window, you have no way of foretelling the result of your action. To be sure, the cat may also escape through the window, but it may just as well crawl under the couch or leap furiously right in your face. The animal of a higher order of life has a much wider choice of action because its sense organs enable it to distinguish so many more details—in other words, because its outside world is incomparably richer. The eyes of the fly can distinguish only the light-filled window and the dark room, but a cat sees a thousand details: the couch, the closet, the dark corner, its pursuer, the window, and so on. It is impossible to predict which of these simultaneous optical stimuli it will react to, and this is why the observer is under the impression that the animal acts by deliberate volition.

The human being presents an even more complicated picture. In most of the things that we humans do, we are not guided solely, as animals are, by our sensory impressions of the moment. Various memory images, the sensory stimuli of past moments, pop up before the mind's eye. These memory images together with the immediate sensory impressions act as co-determinants of our actions. Considerations that link themselves with lightning speed to what we have just perceived lend more weight to one sensory impression, detract from another. The outcome of all these processes is our "decision." How does this decision come into being? We humans believe that we are at liberty to decide freely, in mastery of the situation, after an analysis of all the sensory data perceived through our senses and processed in our brains. It is as if a royal advisory council were presenting recommendations to a king, each member of the council expounding his own opinion, some loudly, in voices resounding with conviction, others in plain words, letting the facts speak for themselves. The king hears them all out and then decides as he deems best, not always in favor of the loudest orator. This is the thesis of the freedom of the will, pet theory of philosophers.

"Freedom of the will" may well turn out to be an illusion, a deceitful mirage conjured up by man's vanity. For all we know, there may be no such king in the realm of the mind, and our "decisions," of which we are so proud, may perhaps be no more free than an animal's— the results of strife among many rival sensory impressions occurring within us and yet completely unknown to us.

There are many arguments in favor of this unglamorous theory. If the conflict among stimuli is resolved by the dominance of one stimulus over all the others, proud Man falls from the lofty summit of free will to the level of an animal which is compelled to react to a certain stimulus in a certain way. If you place a bucket full of water before a group of men, under ordinary circumstances nothing will happen. But if those men have been tormented by thirst for days, so that their tongues cling to their parched palates, they will race for the bucket of water in uncontrolled frenzy—they will turn positively hydrotactic, even as our water fleas turned phototactic when carbon dioxide was squirted into the water in which they swam.

Associations

The stimuli that impinge on our senses are often ephemeral: the tones of a melody reach your ears for an instant; in a crowded street your glance may rest on a strange face for just a few seconds. But such a fleeting contact is sufficient to enable you to recognize that melody or that face if you encounter it again months later.

If you have once enjoyed the fragrance of fine Italian olive oil, a mere whiff of the stuff is enough to recall the experience years later. This means that when you smelled the oil for the first time, a permanent change took place in you. The fragrance of the oil produced a structural change in some cell or group of cells in your brain, which, though it could not be revealed by the most minute examination, is yet a change of an amazingly final character. This structural change manifests itself in your act of recognition when you encounter the same stimulus for a second time. But you can do more than simply recognize the original stimulus. Say that your first experience of olive oil occurred in Italy, and your second encounter takes place in your own kitchen. There is something miraculous about the result. Suddenly, like a haunting ghost from the distant past, far-away Italy looms up about you; you hear the melodious voices of the street peddlers and the shouts of the donkey drivers, you feel the warm sun, you see the colorful Italian street. You remember the pleasant people with whom you shared these moments so many years ago. And all this emerges from the scent of a little oil being heated in your kitchen.

Science calls this remarkable process association. This term signifies that when different senses are stimulated at the same time, delicate cross-connections are produced between the excited areas of the brain. These connections last for months, for years, even for a lifetime. If one of these areas is later excited in the same way, the excitation races along the cross-connections to the other areas and again generates in them the original sensation.

Associations are not the exclusive property of man. They play a most important role for all animals. Perhaps no form of animal life, not even the tiniest and simplest ones, could get along without any associations. But since this amazing revival of the past takes place deep inside your mind, no one else can know anything about it. Your imagination is the only judge of how common this phenomenon is among animals.

Although animals do not give us much information concerning the frequency of association, they do offer us the possibility of studying the associations in their

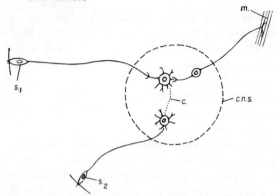

FIG. 55. Diagrammatic representation of the nervous elements which participate in association in the nervous center. *s.₁*, the sensory cell receiving the primary stimulus; *s.₂*, the sensory cell receiving the secondary stimulus; *c.*, connective path; *c.n.s.*, central nervous system; *m.*, muscle.

simplest form. Let us assume, as a simple case, that a stimulus S_1, which always triggers off a definite reflex movement, is accompanied by a second stimulus, S_2, which produces no reaction by itself. Gradually a connection will develop between their respective centers in the interior of the nervous system, permitting S_2 to have a share in the reflex movement (Fig. 55). Now, if we completely suppress S_1 and expose the organism only to S_2, the latter will produce the motor reaction which previously only S_1 could trigger off.

Pavlov made a study of the development of such associations, particularly in dogs. His researches disclosed that if we show a red disk to a dog or let it hear the sound of a whistle every time it is fed, the animal will soon associate the sight of the red disk or the sound of the whistle with food; after a short time it will react to the disk or to the whistle exactly as it would to food. This reaction can be demonstrated. The stimulation of the food starts salivation in the dog's mouth, and the flow of saliva can be measured with precision; soon we find that the saliva begins to drip whenever the animal sees the food or the red disk, or hears the whistle. Associations can be established between the most diverse stimuli. For instance, if you consistently pinch the dog before each feeding, after a time the pinching alone will cause the salivation.

Since we have no access to the sensory world of animals, we have no knowledge of associations other than those that originate from some external stimulus. The case is different with human beings. We have seen that as a result of association with other stimuli, our sensory centers may react, without external stimulation, exactly as they would if they were stimulated by their own sensory cells. The mere idea of a stimulus is often sufficient to produce an effect.

Some of the senses are more likely than others to be affected by associations. Many people are unable to imagine a certain smell or a certain taste; it seems that the lasting associations are the important ones. Almost everyone can recall a dead friend. You see all his familiar movements and gestures, and you hear the sound of his voice, which will never reach your ears again.

Thus we realize that our brains, even when cut off from the outside world, will still convey to us the pale, skeletal residue of previous sensory impressions—like the magic mirror of fairy tales which captures the image of whoever gazes into it and shows the image again to whoever asks to see it. If there were no such inner sense capable of reflecting on all that has entered our minds through the gates of our eyes and ears, aging would be a sad affair indeed. As the cycle of a person's life draws to its end, the sensory powers gradually desert the tired body like withered leaves shaken off a tree by the autumn winds. Eyes and ears become dim and weak, no longer capable of noticing the beauty of this world. But the world of the imagination—the shadow of the world of the senses—permits us to enjoy again all the beauty that was ever ours in life.   ■ ■ ■

INDEX

Available in

ANN ARBOR SCIENCE LIBRARY
OR
ANN ARBOR SCIENCE PAPERBACKS

THE STARS *by W. Kruse and W. Dieckvoss*

THE ANTS *by Wilhelm Goetsch*

THE SENSES *by Wolfgang von Buddenbrock*

LIGHT: VISIBLE AND INVISIBLE *by Eduard Ruechardt*

THE BIRDS *by Oskar and Katharina Heinroth*

EBB AND FLOW: THE TIDES OF EARTH, AIR, AND WATER
by Albert Defant

ANIMAL CAMOUFLAGE *by Adolf Portmann*

PLANET EARTH *by Karl Stumpff*

VIRUS *by Wolfhard Weidel*

THE SUN *by Karl Kiepenheuer*

THE UNIVERSITY OF MICHIGAN PRESS